Advanced Trauma Life Support Course™ for Physicians

This program is dedicated to the care of all victims of trauma.

Published 1989. Third Impression, 1991

Advanced Trauma Life Support™ Student Manual
ISBN 0962037052

Printed in the United States of America

The Role of the Committee on Trauma of the American College of Surgeons

The American College of Surgeons (ACS), founded to improve the care of the surgical patient, has long been a leader in establishing and maintaining the high quality of surgical practice in North America. In accordance with that role, and recognizing that **trauma is a surgical disease**, the ACS Committee on Trauma has worked to establish standards for the care of the trauma patient.

Accordingly, the Committee sponsors and contributes to the continued development of the Advanced Trauma Life Support (ATLS) Course for Physicians. The ATLS course does not present new concepts in the field of trauma care. It does, however, teach well-established treatment methods and approaches trauma care in a systematized manner, presenting to the physician a concise method of establishing assessment and management priorities in the care of the trauma patient.

Revision of the ATLS course content material is conducted every four years by the Subcommittee on ATLS of the ACS Committee on Trauma. Thus the material represents a standard and timely approach to the early care of the trauma patient. By introducing this course and maintaining its high quality, the Committee hopes to provide another instrument by which to reduce the mortality and morbidity related to trauma. **The Committee on Trauma recommends that physicians participating in the ATLS Student Course retake the entire course every four years, in order to maintain both their current status in the ATLS program, and their knowledge of state-of-the-art trauma care.**

American College of Surgeons Committee on Trauma
Erwin R. Thal, MD, FACS
Chairman

Subcommittee on Advanced Trauma Life Support of the American College of Surgeons Committee on Trauma 1987-1988
Max L. Ramenofsky, MD, FACS, Chairman

Charles Aprahamian, MD, FACS
Rea Brown, MD, FACS
Thomas Gennarelli, MD, FACS
Norman McSwain, Jr., MD, FACS
Ernest E. Moore, MD, FACS
Stuart Reynolds, MD, FACS
James Salander, MD, FACS

Jameel Ali, MD, FACS
Paul Collicott, MD, FACS
Brent Krantz, MD, FACS
Kimball Maull, MD, FACS
Herbert Proctor, MD, FACS
Gerald Strauch, MD, FACS

Notice

This edition has been prepared for the Committee on Trauma of the American College of Surgeons by members of the Subcommittee on ATLS, other individual Fellows of the College, and nonsurgical consultants to the Subcommittee who were selected for their special competence in the first hour of trauma care, and for their expertise in medical education. The College believes that those having the responsibility for such patients will find the information valuable. It must be recognized that injured patients present a wide range of complex problems. Accordingly, the authors have presented a concise approach to assessing and managing the multiply injured patient in the first hour. The course presents the physician with knowledge and techniques that are comprehensive and easily adapted to fit his needs. The skills presented in this manual recommend one way to perform each technique. The American College of Surgeons recognizes that there are other acceptable approaches.

Statement on AIDS

The Committee on Trauma of the American College of Surgeons urges all physicians who care for trauma patients to be knowledgeable of the Acquired Immune Deficiency Syndrome (AIDS), take precautionary measures when caring for potential AIDS patients, and be instrumental in establishing or following recommended institutional guidelines. Although a number of documents are available on this subject, information changes with some frequency as more data become available. The Committee on Trauma recommends contacting the Center for Disease Control for the latest information and guidelines.

Contributing Authors

The ACS Committee on Trauma gratefully acknowledges the following individuals for their medical expertise and support in the development of the ATLS course materials.

Jameel Ali, MD, FACS
Professor and Head, Division of General Surgery, Sunnybrook Medical Center, University of Toronto, Toronto, Ontario.

Charles Aprahamian, MD, FACS
Associate Professor of Surgery, Chief of Trauma Service, Medical College of Wisconsin; Director, Institute of Trauma and Emergency Medicine, Milwaukee.

Emidio Bianco, MD, JD
Assistant Chairman, Professional Affairs, Department of Legal Medicine, Armed Forces Institute of Pathology, Washington, DC.

Rea Brown, MD, FACS
Professor of Surgery, McGill University; Director of Surgical Intensive Care Trauma Center, Montreal General Hospital, Montreal.

Carlos Fernandez-Bueno, MD
Assistant Professor of Surgery, Uniformed Services University of the Health Sciences; Chief, Army/Navy Transplant Service, Walter Reed Army Medical Center, Washington, DC.

Paul E. Collicott, MD, FACS
Clinical Assistant Professor of Surgery, University of Nebraska College of Medicine, Omaha, Nebraska; Lincoln, Nebraska.

Frank X. Doto, MS
Professor of Health Education, County College of Morris, Randolph, New Jersey.

Thomas A. Gennarelli, MD, FACS
Associate Professor of Neurosurgery, University of Pennsylvania, Philadelphia.

John H. George, PhD
Physician Liaison, Lincoln General Hospital, Lincoln, Nebraska.

Richard L. Judd, PhD
Executive Dean and Professor of Emergency Medical Sciences, Central Connecticut State University, New Britain, Connecticut.

Brent Krantz, MD, FACS
Chairman, Department of Surgery, Fargo Clinic, Fargo, North Dakota.

Katherine Lane, PhD
Director of Education, Department of Surgery; Assistant Professor of Surgery; Assistant Dean, Clinical Education, State University of New York, Health Sciences, Brooklyn, New York.

Francis G. Lapiana, MD, FACS
Professor of Surgery, Uniformed Services University of the Health Sciences; Director, Ophthalmic, Plastic, Reconstruction, and Orbital Surgery, Walter Reed Army Medical Center, Washington, DC.

Thomas G. Luerssen, MD, FACS
Assistant Professor of Neurosurgery and Pediatrics, University of California San Diego Medical Center, San Diego.

Kimball I. Maull, MD, FACS
Professor and Chairman, Department of Surgery, The University of Tennessee Medical Center at Knoxville, Knoxville, Tennessee.

James A. McGehee, DVM, MS
Assistant Professor of Clinical Surgery and Chief, Veterinary Surgery Division, Department of Laboratory Animal Medicine, Uniformed Services University of the Health Sciences, Bethesda, Maryland.

Norman E. McSwain, Jr., MD, FACS
Professor of Surgery, Director of Trauma Services, Tulane University School of Medicine, New Orleans.

Cynthia L. Meyer, MD
Instructor of Surgery, Uniformed Services University of the Health Sciences; Senior Resident, Otolaryngology Service, Walter Reed Army Medical Center, Washington, DC.

Ernest E. Moore, MD, FACS
Chief, Department of Surgery, Denver General Hospital; Professor and Vice Chairman of Surgery, University of Colorado Health Sciences Center, Denver.

James B. Nichols, DVM, MS
Associate Professor of Clinical Surgery (Affil.), Uniformed Services University of the Health Sciences, Bethesda, Maryland; Administrator, U.S. Air Force Military Training Network, Wiesbaden Regional Medical Center, Wiesbaden, Germany.

Frank Olson, EdD
Professor of Education and Chairman of Secondary Education, Pacific Lutheran University, Tacoma, Washington.

Herbert Proctor, MD, FACS
Professor of Surgery; Head, Trauma Section, University of North Carolina, Chapel Hill, North Carolina.

Max L. Ramenofsky, MD, FACS
Professor of Surgery and Pediatrics, University of Pittsburgh College of Medicine; Director, Pediatric Surgery Training Program and Director, Benedum Pediatric Trauma Program, Children's Hospital of Pittsburgh, Pittsburgh.

Stuart Reynolds, MD, FACS
Chief of Surgery, Northern Montana Hospital, Havre, Montana.

Ronald E. Rosenthal, MD, FACS
Chief, Division of Trauma, Department of Orthopedic Surgery, Long Island Jewish Medical Center, New Hyde Park, New York; Associate Professor Clinical Orthopedic Surgery, State University of New York, Stony Brook, New York.

James M. Salander, MD, FACS
Associate Professor of Surgery, Uniformed Services University of the Health Sciences, Bethesda, Maryland; Chief, Vascular Surgery, Walter Reed Army Medical Center, Washington, DC.

Richard C. Simmonds, DVM, MS
Associate Professor of Surgery and Associate Professor of Physiology; Director, Instructional and Research Support, Uniformed Services University of the Health Sciences, Bethesda, Maryland.

Gerald O. Strauch, MD, FACS
Director, Trauma and Assembly Departments, American College of Surgeons, Chicago; Clinical Professor of Surgery, University of Chicago; Adjunct Professor of Surgery, Northwestern University Medical School, Chicago; Clinical Professor of Surgery, Uniformed Services University of the Health Sciences, F. Hebert School of Medicine, Bethesda, Maryland.

Peter G. Trafton, MD, FACS
Associate Professor, Department of Orthopedics, Brown University; Surgeon in Charge, Division of Trauma, Department of Orthopedics and Rehabilitation, Rhode Island Hospital; Chief of Orthopedic Surgery, Providence Veterans Administration Medical Center, Providence, Rhode Island.

Irvene K. Hughes, RN
Staff, ACS Trauma Department, Administrator, ATLS Programs, Chicago.

Acknowledgements

The ACS Committee on Trauma also gratefully acknowledges the following individuals who reviewed the core medical content for its validity and relevance to private and academic practice.

Doug Davey, MD
Edmonton, Alberta

A. Brent Eastman, MD, FACS
La Jolla, California

Frank E. Ehrlich, MD, FACS
Philadelphia

David V. Feliciano, MD, FACS
Houston

James D. Heckman, MD, FACS
San Antonio, Texas

Howard B. Keith, MD, FACS
Woodward, Oklahoma

Steven J. Kilkenny, MD, FACS
Anchorage, Alaska

Brent Krantz, MD, FACS
Fargo, North Dakota

Anna M. Ledgerwood, MD, FACS
Detroit

Arnold Luterman, MD, FACS
Mobile, Alabama

Gerald McCullough, MD, FACS
Norman, Oklahoma

David Mulder, MD, FACS
Montreal

Lawrence H. Pitts, MD, FACS
San Francisco

Richard R. Price, MD, FACS
Salt Lake City

Marleta Reynolds, MD, FACS
Chicago, Illinois

Arnold Sladen, MD, FACS
Pittsburgh, Pennsylvania

Luther M. Strayer, III, MD
Park Ridge, Illinois

Joseph J. Tepas, MD, FACS
Jacksonville, Florida

Raymond L. Warpeha, MD, FACS
Maywood, Illinois

John A. Weigelt, MD, FACS
Dallas

Robert J. White, MD, FACS
Cleveland

Fremont P. Wirth, MD, FACS
Savannah, Georgia

Table of Contents

Appendices

American College of Surgeons

ATLS
Core Course Content

Course Overview, Concept, and History

Trauma is the leading cause of death in the first four decades of life in the United States, surpassed only by cancer and atherosclerosis as the cause of death in all age groups. The number of disabling injuries and trauma-related deaths occurring each year is staggering; the cost of human suffering and life, incalculable.

In the 1- to 34-year age group, trauma accounts for more deaths in the United States than all other diseases combined. Fifty million injuries occur annually, ten million of which are disabling. For every death from trauma, there are two permanent disabilities. Annually, over 80,000 people sustain permanently disabling injuries of the brain or spinal cord. The incidence of major trauma is 1,000 per million American population annually. Twelve percent of all hospital beds are occupied by trauma patients. More than 140,000 deaths occur annually from injuries. However, unlike mortality from many serious diseases in the United States, the mortality from injuries is increasing each year. The costs for trauma care in the United States are staggering. Injuries account for one of the most expensive health problems, costing $75 billion to $100 billion annually, directly and indirectly. However, injury research receives less than two cents out of every federal dollar expended for research on health problems.

Trauma, without respect for age, swift in onset and slow in recovery, presents many pitfalls for the responsible physician caring for the trauma patient. Trauma is merciless in its lethal and mangling pathways through our young and potentially productive members of society. Prevention is the best cure, but when prevention fails, the physician must be sufficiently knowledgeable to meet the injured patient's needs and reduce the mortality and morbidity of trauma.

Death from trauma has a trimodal distribution. The **first peak of death** is within seconds to minutes of injury. Deaths occurring during this period are usually due to lacerations of the brain, brain stem, high spinal cord, heart, aorta, or other large vessels. Only a few of these patients can be salvaged and then only in large urban areas where rapid emergency transport is available. The **second death peak** occurs within minutes to a few hours after injury. Some have referred to this period as the **golden hour** for the critically injured. **The primary focus of the Advanced Trauma Life Support Course is on this first hour of trauma management, when rapid assessment and resuscitation can be carried out to reduce this second peak of trauma deaths.** Deaths occuring during this period are usually due to subdural and epidural hematomas, hemopneumothorax, ruptured spleen, lacerations of the liver, pelvic fractures, or multiple injuries associated with significant blood loss. The fundamental principles of trauma care learned in this course can be best applied to these patients. The **third death peak** occurs several days or weeks after the initial injury, and is almost always due to sepsis and organ failure. Therefore, the first person to assess the patient can affect the final outcome.

As with most critical illnesses, the quality of the initial assessment and management of the severely injured patient influences the final outcome. Trauma cuts across the entire field of medicine, requiring the physician to have a broad knowledge base of treatment principles and an appreciation for multiple varieties of injury. An organized, consistent approach to the trauma patient affords an optimal outcome.

Properly trained ambulance personnel and adequately equipped vehicles result only from the efforts of physicians who demand to receive their patients in the best possible condition. Standing orders and established protocols for trauma patients that allow properly trained and certified personnel to initiate life-saving procedures are a necessity in the absence of a physician.

Before 1980 the delivery of trauma care by physicians in the United States was inconsistent; national standards for trauma care were nonexistent; and a standardized, national trauma program to train physicians how to care for the trauma patient in the first hour did not exist. In February 1976, a tragic accident occurred which ultimately resulted in conceptualization of the Advanced Trauma Life Support Course. A Nebraskan surgeon, piloting his small fixed-wing plane to Lincoln, crashed in a wooded area. The surgeon sustained serious injuries; three of his children, critical injuries; and one child, minor injuries. His wife was killed instantly. Reportedly, the initial care received by the father and his children was tragically inadequate and far below today's minimum standards of trauma care. As a result of this tragedy and recognizing the need for improved trauma care in the small community hospital, the surgeon approached the staff at the Lincoln Medical Education Foundation (LMEF) and Southeast Nebraska Emergency Medical Services with an educational concept. In his words: " When I can provide better care in the field with limited resources than what my children and I received at the primary care facility — there is something wrong with the system and the system has to be changed. "

Other private-practice surgeons and physicians in Nebraska agreed and supported his concept. They identified the need for training in advanced trauma life support using a combined educational format of lecture presentation and associated skill demonstration and practicum. In response to this expressed need, the LMEF Physician's Committee on Trauma developed a prototype Advanced Trauma Life Support (ATLS) Course for physicians. The first ATLS Course was field-tested in conjunction with Southeast Nebraska Emergency Medical Services in 1978.

After revisions by the University of Nebraska Medical Center and the LMEF Physician's Committee on Trauma, the American College of Surgeons Committee on Trauma adopted the ATLS Course in 1979. Further revisions were made in the essential course content to provide a standardized national trauma program.

Based on the original concept, this course is primarily targeted at the physician who does **not** deal with major trauma on a day-to-day basis, who must evaluate and manage the seriously injured patient during the period immediately after injury. However, over the ensuing years since its inception, the course content is now recognized and accepted as beneficial to all physicians caring for the trauma patient.

Based on well-established objectives of trauma management, this course is intended to provide the physician with one acceptable method of immediate management, and the basic knowledge and skills necessary to:

1. Assess the patient's condition rapidly and accurately.

2. Resuscitate and stabilize the patient on a priority basis.

3. Determine if a patient's needs will likely exceed a facility's capabilities.

4. Arrange for the patient's interhospital transfer.

5. Assure that optimum care is provided each step of the way.

The Advanced Trauma Life Support Course emphasizes the first hour of initial assessment and primary management of the trauma patient, starting at the point and time of injury and continuing through initial assessment; life-saving intervention; re-evaluation; stabilization; and where needed, transfer to another health care facility. The course will consist of pre- and postcourse tests, lectures, case presentations, discussions, and development of life-saving manipulative skills, practical laboratory experience, and a performance proficiency evaluation. Upon completion of this course the physician should feel confident in implementing the basic trauma skills taught in the ATLS Course.

The Committee on Trauma of the American College of Surgeons gratefully acknowledges these organizations for their time and efforts in developing and field testing the Advanced Trauma Life Support concept: The Lincoln Medical Education Foundation, Southeast Nebraska Emergency Medical Services, The University of Nebraska College of Medicine, and the Nebraska State Committee on Trauma of the American College of Surgeons. The Committee on Trauma has borrowed extensively from their experience and material. We are indebted to those Nebraska physicians who encouraged the development of this course, and to those Lincoln Area Mobile Heart Team nurses who shared their time and ideas to help build the ATLS Course.

The Committee on Trauma of the American College of Surgeons hopes that through the applications of the skills taught in the Advanced Trauma Life Support Course, a significant reduction in trauma morbidity and subsequent mortality will be accomplished. The establishment of a minimum standard of care in the early assessment and management of the trauma patient most assuredly will bring this about. Through the dedicated efforts of health care professionals, this worthy goal can be achieved.

Bibliography

1. Committee on Trauma Research, Commission on Life Sciences, National Research Council, and the Institute of Medicine: **Injury in America.** Washington, DC, National Academy Press, 1985.

2. Trunkey, Donald D: The Value of Trauma Centers. **ACS Bulletin** 1982;67:10, 5 - 7,

3. Trunkey, Donald D: Trauma. **Scientific American** 1983; 249:28-35.

American College of Surgeons

General Course Objectives

The purpose of this course is to orient physicians to the initial assessment and management of the trauma victim. In general, the content and skills presented in the materials are designed to assist physicians in providing the **first hour** of emergency care for the trauma patient. Therefore, this course represents the minimum information necessary to manage the trauma patient in the first hour.

Upon completion of the Advanced Trauma Life Support Course, the physician participant will be able to :

A. Demonstrate concepts and principles of primary and secondary patient asessment.

B. Establish management priorities in a trauma situation.

C. Initiate primary and secondary management necessary within the first hour of emergency care for acute life- threatening emergencies.

D. Demonstrate, in a given simulated clinical and surgical skill practicum, the following skills used in the initial assessment and management of patients with multiple injuries:

   1. Primary and secondary assessment of a moulage victim with multiple injuries.

   2. Orotracheal and nasotracheal intubation on adult and infant manikins.

   3. Cricothyroidotomy.

   4. Initiation of central intravenous lifelines with central venous pressure monitoring.

   5. Administration of intravenous fluid therapy in conjunction with different types of shock.

   6. Venous cutdown.

   7. Application, inflation, deflation, and removal of a pneumatic antishock garment.

   8. Pleural decompression via needle thoracentesis and chest tube insertion.

   9. Pericardiocentesis.

   10. Peritoneal lavage.

   11. Roentgenographic identification of cervical spine injuries.

   12. Cervical spine and long spine immobilization and stabilization prior to patient transfer.

   13. Application of extremity splints.

Chapter 1:
Initial Assessment and Management

Objectives:

Upon completion of this topic, the physician will be able to demonstrate an ability to apply the principles of emergency medical care to the multiply injured patient. Specifically, the physician will be able to:

A. Identify the correct sequence of priorities of emergency medical care to be followed in assessing the multiply injured patient.

B. Outline the primary and secondary evaluation surveys to be used in assessing the multiply injured patient.

C. Identify and discuss the key components of and rationale for obtaining the patient's history and the history of the trauma incident.

D. Explain guidelines and techniques to be used in the initial resuscitative and definitive-care phases of treatment of the multiply injured patient.

E. Conduct an initial assessment and management survey on a simulated multiply injured patient, using the correct sequence of priorities and explaining management techniques for primary treatment and stabilization.

**Chapter 1:
Initial
Assessment
and
Management**

I. Introduction

The prioritized assessment and management procedures reviewed in this chapter are identified as sequential steps in order of their importance for purpose of clarity. However, these steps are frequently accomplished **simultaneously.** For example, while conducting a rapid assessment of the patient's respiratory, circulatory, and neurologic status, the patient's history and events related to the injury must also be obtained.

The written description of these steps does not allow for this simultaneous integration, and artificially separates these integrated activities. Although each step is important, some require immediate attention as life-threatening injuries are identified. For example, the patient's response to the question "What happened?" can provide information about his airway, breathing, and neurologic status. Simultaneously, the examiner can assess the patient's pulse, skin color, and capillary refilling time. As a result of assessing and managing the patient in this manner, important information concerning the patient's status has been obtained simultaneously in the first 30 seconds of patient contact.

The importance of obtaining the patient's history and history of injury are emphasized in this chapter. Halsted's philosophy relates that obtaining patient and event histories represents 90% of the diagnostic evaluation. This philosophical approach is used when evaluating and managing the trauma patient. If complete histories are not obtained, major injuries may be missed or pre-existing medical factors that may compromise the patient's outcome or prolong the hospital stay may be overlooked. **The physician must understand the kinematics of trauma and integrate this knowledge with the trauma-producing episode. Prehospital personnel are the primary source of this important component of the patient's history.**

II. Establishing Assessment and Management Priorities

Patients are assessed and treatment priorities established based on their injuries and the stability of their vital signs, and on the mechanism of the traumatic incident. In an emergency involving a critical injury, logical sequential treatment priorities must be established based on the overall patient assessment. The patient's vital functions must be assessed quickly and efficiently. Patient management must consist of a rapid primary evaluation, resuscitation of vital functions, a more detailed secondary assessment, and finally, the initiation of definitive care.

A. Primary Survey: ABCs

During the **primary survey**, life-threatening conditions are identified and management is begun **simultaneously.**

1. **A**—Airway maintenance with cervical spine control
2. **B**—Breathing and ventilation
3. **C**—Circulation with hemorrhage control
4. **D**—Disability: Neurologic status
5. **E**—Exposure: Completely undress the patient

B. Resuscitation Phase

Shock management is initiated, management of patient oxygenation is re-assessed, and hemorrhage control is re-evaluated. The life-threatening conditions identified in the primary survey are constantly reassessed, as management is continued. Tissue aerobic metabolism is assured by perfusion of all tissue with well-oxygenated red blood cells. Replacement of lost vascular volume with warmed crystalloid fluids and blood is begun, as are other modalities of shock therapy. A urinary catheter and nasogastric tube may also be inserted during this phase, if their use is not contraindicated.

C. Secondary Survey

The secondary survey does not begin until the primary survey (ABCs) has been completed and the resuscitation phase (management of other life-threatening conditions) has begun.

The secondary survey is a head-to-toe evaluation of the trauma patient, which includes vital sign assessment—blood pressure, pulse, respirations, and temperature. This in-depth evaluation employs the look, listen, and feel techniques, evaluating the body by regions. Each region (head, neck, chest, abdomen, extremities, and neurologic) is examined individually. The stethoscope is used over each body cavity and major vessel area. The hands palpate for bony defects and other abnormalities. A neurologic examination, including the Glasgow Coma Scale, completes the secondary assessment. Chest and cervical spine roentgenograms are obtained early as soon as practical. These films take precedence over subsequent roentgenographic evaluation.

Special procedures required for patient assessment, such as peritoneal lavage, radiologic evaluation, and laboratory studies, are also conducted in this phase. Assessment of the eyes, ears, nose, mouth, rectum, and pelvis should not be neglected. This examination can be easily described as "tubes and fingers in every orifice."

D. Definitive-Care Phase

In the definitive-care phase, all the patient's injuries are managed. This phase includes comprehensive management, fracture stabilization, and any necessary operative intervention, as well as stabilization of the patient in preparation for appropriate transfer to a facility that can provide a higher level of medical care.

The omission of any of these steps during assessment or treatment of the injured patient can result in unnecessary disability or death. Primarily because prehospital care personnel have improved their knowledge and skills, many of these problems will have been addressed before the patient arrives in the emergency department. Observations made by prehospital personnel concerning the patient and mechanism of injury must be considered while reassessing the patient's condition in the emergency department. Changes in the patient's vital signs, respiratory and circulatory status, and neurologic functions can be expected.

When triage requires identification of patients who must be transported to a trauma center, the **Interhospital Triage Criteria** is a useful reference. (See Chapter 12—Stabilization and Transport.)

E. Pediatric Priorities

Priorities for the care of the pediatric patient are basically the same as for adults. Although the quantities of blood and fluids, the size of the child, degree of heat loss, and injury patterns may differ, assessment and priorities are the same. Specific problems of the pediatric trauma patient are addressed in Chapter 10. The Pediatric Trauma Score is helpful in identifying those severely injured patients who should be transported to a trauma center. (See Appendix B—Pediatric Triage and Injury Scoring.)

F. Triage

Triage is a sorting of patients based on need for treatment. A group of injured patients can be satisfactorily evaluated and resuscitation begun with the help of nurses and EMT personnel (when available). Treatment is rendered based on the ABC priorities (Airway with cervical spine control, Breathing, and Circulation with hemorrhage control) as previously outlined.

Two types of triage situations usually exist.

1. The number of patients and the severity of their injuries do **not** exceed the ability of the facility to render care. In this situation, patients with life-threatening problems and those sustaining multiple-system injuries are treated first.

2. The number of patients and the severity of their injuries **exceed** the capability of the facility and staff. In this situation, those patients with the greatest chance of survival, with the least expenditure of time, equipment, supplies, and personnel, are managed first.

III. Priority Plan—Treatment and Management

A. Primary Survey

1. Airway and cervical spine

The upper airway should be assessed to ascertain patency. Initial attempts to establish a patent airway include the chin lift or jaw thrust maneuver, or removal of foreign debris. Specific attention should be given to the possibility of cervical spine fractures. Excessive movement of the cervical spine can convert a fracture without neurological damage into a fracture-dislocation with neurologic injury. Therefore, the patient's head and neck should not be hyperextended or hyperflexed to establish or maintain an airway.

Remember: Assume a cervical spine fracture in any patient with multisystem trauma, especially with a blunt injury above the clavicle. Based on the history of the trauma incident, the loss of integrity of the cervical spine should be suspected. Neurological examination alone does not rule out a cervical spine injury. The integrity of the bony components of the cervical spine can be initially assessed by visualizing all seven cervical vertebrae, including the C-7 to T-1 interspace, on a crosstable lateral cervical spine roentgenogram or a swimmer's view. However, the lateral cervical spine radiograph does not rule out all cervical spine injuries. Based on clinical judgment, immobilization procedures should be maintained until serial roentgenograms of the cervical spine and neurosurgical or orthopedic consultation are obtained.

2. Breathing

The patient's chest should be exposed to adequately assess ventilatory exchange. Airway patency does not assure adequate ventilation. Adequate air exchange is necessary, in addition to an open airway, for sufficient oxygenation. Until the patient is stable, ventilation should be accomplished with a bag-valve device connected to a mask or endotracheal tube. If the bag-valve mask device is used, the two-man technique should be employed. (See Chapter 2–Airway Management and Ventilation.) Adequate oxygenation and ventilation of the trauma patient must include the delivery of adequate volume and inspired concentrations of oxygen (eg, FIO_2 greater than 0.85). **This cannot be accomplished with nasal prongs or a simple face mask.** Three traumatic conditions that most often compromise ventilation are: tension pneumothorax, open pneumothorax, and large flail chest with pulmonary contusion. A respiratory rate of greater than 20/minute should alert the examiner to the possibility of respiratory compromise.

3. Circulation

a. Blood volume and cardiac output

Among the causes of early postinjury deaths in the hospital that are amenable to effective treatment, hemorrhage is predominant. Hypotension following injury must be assumed to be hypovolemic in origin until proved otherwise. Rapid and accurate assessment of the injured patient's hemodynamic status is therefore essential. Three elements of observation yield key information within seconds. They are state of consciousness, skin color, and pulse.

1) State of consciousness

When blood volume is reduced by half or more, cerebral perfusion is critically impaired, and unconsciousness results. Conversely, a conscious patient can be presumed to have at least enough blood volume to maintain cerebral perfusion.

2) Skin color

A patient with pink skin, especially in the face and extremities, is rarely critically hypovolemic following injury. Conversely, the ashen, gray skin of the face and the white skin of blood-drained extremities are ominous signs of hypovolemia. These latter signs usually indicate a blood volume loss of at least 30 percent if hypovolemia is the cause.

3) Pulse

Full, slow, regular peripheral pulses are welcome signs in the injured patient. The physician will usually check an easily accessible central pulse initially, and femoral or carotid pulses signify coordinated cardiac action and at least 50 percent of residual blood volume. Rapid, thready pulses are early signs of hypovolemia, but may have other causes as well. An irregular pulse is usually a warning of cardiac impairment. Absent central pulses at more than one site, without local injuries or other factors which preclude accurate palpation of pulses, signify the need for immediate resuscitative action to restore depleted blood volume, effective cardiac output, or both, within seconds or minutes, if death is to be avoided.

b. Bleeding

External, exsanguinating hemorrhage should be identified and controlled in the primary survey. Rapid blood loss is managed by direct pressure on the wound. Pneumatic splints may also help control hemorrhage. The use of hemostats is extremely time- consuming and dangerous. **Tourniquets ordinarily should not be used** because they can produce anaerobic metabolism as well as increased blood loss if incorrectly applied. Occult hemorrhage into the thoracic or abdominal cavities, into the muscle body surrounding a fracture, or as a result of penetrating injury, can account for a major blood loss. Abdominal or lower-extremity hemorrhage can be controlled or reduced significantly with the application and inflation of the pneumatic antishock garment.

4. Brief neurologic evaluation (disability)

A rapid neurologic evaluation is performed at the end of the primary survey. This neurologic evaluation establishes the patient's level of consciousness and pupillary size and reaction.

The AVPU method describes the patient's level of consciousness.

A—**A**lert
V—Responds to **V**ocal stimuli
P—Responds to **P**ainful stimuli
U—**U**nresponsive

A more detailed quantitative neurologic examination, ie, the Glasgow Coma Scale, should be included in the secondary survey. Changes in the patient's neurologic condition may indicate intracranial pathology or decreased oxygenation of the central nervous system.

A decrease in the level of consciousness may indicate decreased cerebral oxygenation and/or perfusion. Such a change indicates a need for immediate re-evaluation of the patient's oxygenation, ventilation, and perfusion status.

5. Exposure

The patient should be completely undressed to facilitate thorough examination and assessment.

B. Resuscitation

1. Supplemental **oxygen therapy** is instituted for all trauma patients, preferably via a mask/reservoir device, to achieve an FIO_2 of greater than 0.85.

2. A minimum of **two large-caliber intravenous catheters** (IV's) (#16-gauge or larger) should be established. When initiating the intravenous lines, blood should be drawn for type and crossmatch, and for baseline hematologic and chemical studies.

   Vigorous intravenous fluid therapy should be initiated with a balanced salt solution. The maximum rate of fluid administration is determined by the internal diameter of the catheter and inversely by its length, not by the vein in which the catheter is placed. Initiation of peripheral intravenous lines and/or cutdowns is safer and less complicated than central lines.

   The shocklike state associated with trauma is most often hypovolemic in nature. After two to three liters of balanced salt solution have been administered, type-specific blood may be used as necessary while blood is being prepared. If type-specific blood is not available, consideration should be given to the use of low-titer type-O blood. For life-threatening blood loss, the use of unmatched, type-specific blood is preferred over type-O blood. Whole blood should be used when available. Hypovolemic shock is **not** treated by vasopressors, steroids, or sodium bicarbonate.

3. Adequate resuscitation is best assessed by the quantitative improvement of physiologic parameters, ie, ventilatory rate, pulse, blood pressure, pulse pressure, arterial blood gases (ABGs), and urinary output, rather than the qualitative assessment that is done in the primary survey. Actual values should be obtained as soon as practical after completing the primary sur-vey.

4. Careful **electrocardiographic (ECG) monitoring** of all trauma patients is required. Dysrhythmias, including unexplained tachycardia, atrial fibrillation, premature ventricular contractions, and ST segment changes, may indicate cardiac contusion. Electromechanical dissociation (EMD) may indicate cardiac tamponade, tension pneumothorax, and/or profound hypovolemia. When bradycardia, aberrant conduction, and premature beats are present, hypoxia and hypoperfusion should be suspected immediately. Hypothermia will also produce these dysrhythmias.

5. The placement of **urinary and gastric catheters** should now be considered. Urethral transection and cribriform plate fractures, respectively, contraindicate insertion.

   For male victims of blunt trauma resulting in suspected urethral transection, insertion of a urinary catheter **should not be attempted** before an examination of the rectum and genitalia has been performed. Urinary catheter insertion, without a preceding urethrogram, is usually contraindicated if there is 1) blood at the meatus, 2) blood in the scrotum, and 3) the prostate cannot be palpated or is high-riding.

If the cribriform plate is fractured, the nasogastric tube may be inserted unintentionally into the intracranial cavity. Therefore, in cases of blunt head trauma, nonclotting blood from the ears, nose, or mouth should be evaluated using the "halo" or "double-ring" test **before** insertion of the nasogastric tube. (See Chapter 6—Head Trauma.)

Remember: Airway maintenance, cardiopulmonary resuscitation, and other life-saving modalities for patient care should be initiated when the problem is identified, rather than after the primary survey. After the primary survey and resuscitation phase, the evaluating physician frequently has enough information to indicate the need to transfer the patient to another facility. This transfer process should be initiated immediately by administrative personnel, while additional patient care and evaluation are being managed by the examining physician. The receiving physician should be contacted, and the appropriate mode of transportation identified and mobilized with the proper personnel and equipment.

C. Secondary Survey

1. Head

The secondary survey begins with evaluation of the head and identification of all related and significant injuries. The eyes should be re-evaluated for pupillary size, fundi for hemorrhages, lens for dislocation, conjunctiva for hemorrhages and any penetrating injuries. In addition, assess for the presence of contact lenses and remove them before edema occurs. Do a quick visual confrontation examination of both eyes by having the patient read either a Snelling Chart or words on the side of an intravenous container. This procedure frequently identifies optic injuries not otherwise apparent. (See Appendix A—Ocular Trauma.)

2. Maxillofacial trauma

Maxillofacial trauma not associated with airway obstruction should be treated only after the patient is completely stabilized and is not suffering from any other major life-threatening injuries. Adequate treatment can be initiated within seven to ten days of the injury, although earlier treatment may be instituted as the patient's condition permits.

Patients with midfacial fractures may have a fracture of the cribriform plate. For these patients, gastric intubation should be performed via the oral route or through a soft nasopharyngeal airway, rather than nasally.

3. Cervical spine/neck

All patients with maxillofacial trauma produced by blunt injury should be presumed to have a cervical spine fracture, and the neck should be protected until injury is ruled out. Examination of the neck includes both visual inspection and palpation. **The absence of neurological deficit or pain does not rule out injury to the cervical spine. Such an injury should be presumed present until ruled out by adequate roentgenographic examination.**

Patients wearing any type of sports helmet should have their head and neck held in a neutral position while the helmet is removed. During this two-person procedure, inline manual immobilization is applied from below, and the helmet is expanded laterally. Inline manual immobilization is then re-established from above, and the patient is adequately immobilized.

In penetrating trauma, wounds that extend through the platysma should **not** be manually explored in the emergency department. This type of injury requires surgical evaluation. Nonoperative measures performed by a surgeon include observation, arteriography, bronchoscopy, esophagoscopy, and esophagography.

4. Chest

Visual evaluation of the chest, both anterior and posterior, will identify sucking chest injuries and perhaps a large flail segment. A complete evaluation of the chest wall requires palpation of the entire chest cage, feeling each rib and the clavicles individually. Blunt sternal pressure may be painful if any attached ribs are fractured. Contusions and hematomas of the chest wall should alert the physician to the possibility of more occult injury.

Evaluation of the internal structures is done with the stethoscope, followed by a roentgenogram of the chest. Breath sounds are auscultated high on the anterior chest for pneumothorax and at the posterior bases for hemothorax. Auscultatory findings may be difficult to evaluate in the noisy emergency department. Distant heart sounds and distended neck veins may indicate cardiac tamponade. However, neck veins may be not be distended because of associated hypovolemia. A narrow pulse pressure may be the only reliable indication of cardiac tamponade. Of the five major signs, decreased breath sounds may be the only indication of a tension pneumothorax and the need to initiate chest decompression.

5. Abdomen

Any abdominal injury is potentially dangerous and must be diagnosed and treated aggressively. The specific diagnosis is not as important as the fact that an abdominal injury exists, and surgical intervention may be needed. Initial examination of the abdomen may not be representative of the patient's condition one to several hours later. Close observation and frequent re-evaluation of the abdomen is important in management of blunt abdominal trauma. A change in the patient's overall condition or progression of abdominal pathology may alter these findings over time.

When intra-abdominal hemorrhage is suspected, particularly when associated with shock, **properly applied** pneumatic antishock trousers may slow continued blood loss. Once initiated, this indirect pressure on the hemorrhage site can be beneficial while the patient is en route to the operating room or to a referral hospital. **The pneumatic antishock garment is not designed to supplant volume resuscitation.** (See Chapter 3– Shock.)

Patients with neurological injury, impaired sensorium secondary to alcohol or drugs, or equivocal abdominal findings should be considered candidates for peritoneal lavage. Fractures of the pelvis or the lower rib cage may also hinder adequate diagnostic examination of the abdomen.

6. Rectum

A rectal examination is an essential part of the secondary survey. Specifically, the physician should assess for the presence of blood within the bowel lumen, a high-riding prostate, the presence of pelvic fractures, the integrity of the rectal wall, and the quality of the sphincter tone.

7. Fractures

Extremities should be visually evaluated for contusions or deformity. Palpation of the bones with rotational or three-point pressure, checking for tenderness, crepitation, or abnormal movements along the shaft, helps identify fractures where alignment has been maintained. Anterior to posterior pressure with the heels of the hands on both anterior superior iliac spines and the symphysis pubis can identify pelvic fractures. In addition, all peripheral pulses should be assessed and their presence or absence documented, along with neurologic findings.

Thoracic and lumbar spinal fractures must be considered based on physical findings and mechanism(s) of injury. Other injuries may mask the physical findings of spinal injuries, which may go unsuspected unless the physician obtains appropriate roentgenograms.

8. Neurologic

A comprehensive neurological examination includes not only motor and sensory evaluation of the extremities, but also re-evaluation of the patient's level of consciousness and pupils. A numerical evaluation such as the Glasgow Coma Scale facilitates detection of early changes.

Any evidence of paralysis or paresis suggests major injury to the spinal column or peripheral nervous system. Immobilization of the **entire** patient, using short or long spine boards and a semirigid cervical collar, must be established first. Patient transport to a definitive-care facility requires the same type of adequate immobilization.

A neurosurgeon should treat acute epidural and subdural hematomas, depressed skull fractures, and other intracranial injuries. Changes in intracranial status may be associated with alterations in the level of consciousness. If a patient with a head injury deteriorates neurologically, management and treatment priorities may change. Oxygenation and perfusion of the brain and the adequacy of ventilation should be reassessed. If these parameters are unchanged, intracranial surgical intervention may be indicated. In a community where a neurosurgeon is not available, patients with signs and symptoms of neurologic deterioration should be considered for immediate transfer. A telephone consultation is recommended.

D. Definitive Care

The interhospital triage criteria helps determine the level, pace, and intensity of initial management of the multiply injured patient. It takes into account the patient's physiologic status, obvious anatomic injury, mechanism of injury, concurrent diseases, and factors that may alter the patient's prognosis. Emergency department and surgical personnel should use these criteria to determine if the patient requires transfer to a facility capable of providing more specialized care. (See Chapter 12–Stabilization and Transport.)

IV. Re-evaluate the Patient

The trauma patient should be **re-evaluated** continuously so that any new signs and symptoms are not overlooked. As initial life-threatening injuries are managed, other equally life-threatening problems may become apparent, and less severe injuries or underlying medical problems may become evident. A high index of suspicion and constant alertness facilitate early diagnosis and management.

Continuous monitoring of vital signs and urinary output is essential. For the adult patient, maintenance of a urinary output of 50 ml/hour is desirable. In the pediatric patient over one year of age, an output of 1 ml/kg/hour should be adequate. Arterial blood gas and central cardiac monitoring devices should be employed for all critical patients.

V. History

A. Patient

The patient's pertinent past history must be assessed; the "AMPLE" history is a useful mneumonic.

A—Allergies
M—Medications currently taken
P—Past illnesses
L—Last meal
E—Events/environment related to the injury

B. Mechanism of Injury

A history of the injury or examination of the injury-producing mechanism is very helpful in identifying specific types of injuries. Injury types can be classified according to the direction and amount of energy force. The energy wave extends away from the point of impact in blunt trauma, and laterally from the missile pathway in penetrating trauma.

It is important to recognize that a temporary cavity forms as a result of both types of energy transmission. The examiner must realize that because of the extreme elasticity of the body tissues, the extent of such trauma is not visualized when the patient is first seen in the emergency department. Intrusion into the body cavity occurs even in blunt trauma.

1. Blunt trauma

The severity of injury varies according to the amount of energy transferred from an object to the human body. The automobile accounts for a major portion of severe blunt trauma, and is exemplified in this chapter. However, the physician must also understand the injuries associated with falls, and motorcycle and bicycle trauma.

The direction of impact determines the pattern of injuries. Prehospital personnel should describe the appearance of the vehicle and the damage sustained to the passenger compartment. The occupant usually is injured in the same projection of the car. Because the body's elastic tissue rebounds to its original position, and the metal of the car does not, the deformation of the car can be used to gauge the damage to the patient. Restraining devices, such as seat belts, significantly reduce or prevent many types of injuries. Body cavity injuries are produced by compression and deceleration.

With this information, the physician can judge what portion of the body absorbed the greatest transfer of energy, and what injury patterns are likely in the affected cavities.

a. A frontal impact with a bent steering wheel, knee imprint on the dashboard, and bull's-eye fracture of the windshield should alert the examining physician to the potential for cervical spine injuries, central flail chest, myocardial contusion, pneumothorax, fractured spleen or liver, and posterior fracture-dislocation of the hip.

b. A side impact may cause contralateral neck sprain or cervical fracture, lateral flail chest, pneumothorax, acceleration injury to the aorta, fractured spleen or liver (depending upon the side of impact), and fractured pelvis or acetabulum.

c. Rear-impact collisions can result in neck injuries (ie, cervical strain). Usually there is a frontal-impact component as well because the occupant is projected into the steering wheel.

d. Ejection from a vehicle can result in multiple injuries, including a cervical spine fracture, depending on which part of the body impacted first. The risk of injury increases by 300% when the occupant is ejected from the vehicle.

2. Penetrating trauma

Two factors determine the type of injury and subsequent management.

a. The **region** of the body sustaining the injury determines the potential for specific organ injury.

b. The **transfer** of energy determine the injury itself. The **velocity** of the missile and its mass further determines the amount of energy dissipated. The **distance** from the source is important to identify the amount of energy dissipated before impact with the patient. Energy transfer is determined by the **rate** or **change in speed**, or energy loss while the missile is inside the patient's body.

The frontal impact areas of the missile determines the number of tissue particles impacted, which in turn (along with the tissue density and elasticity) determines the rate of energy exchange. Tumble, fragmentation, and deformation modify the frontal impact area and change the amount and rate of exchange of energy from the missile to the body.

The amount of energy itself is determined by this formula:

$$KE = \frac{MV^2}{2}$$

KE = Kinetic energy
M = Mass
V = Velocity

For most penetrating injuries, the speed of the missile is the most important factor in determining energy.

3. Burns

Burns are significant because of the thermal injury to the skin, as well as smoke inhalation and heat injury to the lungs, carbon monoxide inhalation, and effects of any chemicals involved. Thermal injuries may also be associated with blunt trauma and fractures resulting from an explosion, falling debris, or the patient's attempt to escape the fire.

4. Hypothermia and cold injuries

Acute or chronic reduction of the temperature without adequate protection against heat loss produces either local or generalized hypothermic injuries. Loss of heat into the external environment may occur at moderate temperatures (15 to 20 degrees centigrade) when wet clothes, decreased activity, or vasodilatation caused by alcohol or drugs compromises the patient's ability to conserve heat.

Patients may also become hypothermic during resuscitation in the emergency department, with the rapid administration of room temperature fluids. Control of the patient's body temperature during the resuscitation phase is an important adjunct.

5. Hazardous environment

Chemicals, toxins, and radiation can produce a variety of cutaneous, pulmonary, cardiac, or internal organ derangement. These chemicals can present a hazard not only to patients but to health care providers as well. When such injuries occur, the physician must identify the specific substance involved and its potential for injury. Frequently, the physician's only means of preparation is to have knowledge of the general principles of management of such agents and immediate access to the Regional Poison Control Center.

VI. Disaster

Disasters frequently overwhelm local and regional resources. Plans for management of such conditions must be evaluated and rehearsed frequently to enhance the possibility of significant salvage of injured patients.

VII. Records and Legal Considerations

A. Records

Meticulous record-keeping is very important. Often more than one physician cares for the patient. Precise records are essential to evaluate the patient's needs and clinical status. Do not rely solely on memory.

Medical-legal problems arise frequently, and precise records are helpful for all concerned. Chronologic reporting with flow sheets helps both the attending physician and any other consulting physician to quickly assess changes in the patient's condition.

B. Consent for Treatment

Consent is sought before treatment for obvious reasons. In life-threatening emergencies, the necessary treatment should be given first and formal consent obtained later.

C. Forensic Evidence

If trauma due to criminal activity is suspected, the personnel caring for the patient must preserve the evidence. All items, such as bullets and clothing, must be saved for law enforcement personnel. Entrance and exit wounds should be identified and documented.

VIII. Summary

The injured patient must be evaluated rapidly and thoroughly. The physician must develop priorities for the patient. Treatment priorities must be considered in the overall management of the patient, so no steps in the process are omitted. An adequate patient history and accounting of the incident is also important in evaluating and managing the trauma patient.

Evaluation and care are divided into four phases.

A. Primary Survey–Assessment of ABCs

1. Airway and cervical spine control
2. Breathing
3. Circulation with hemorrhage control
4. Disability: Brief neurological evaluation
5. Exposure: Completely undress the patient

B. Resuscitation

1. Shock management–intravenous lines, Ringer's lactate
2. The management of life-threatening problems identified in the primary survey is continued.
3. Electrocardiographic monitoring

C. Secondary Survey–Total Evaluation of the Patient

1. Head and skull
2. Maxillofacial injuries
3. Neck
4. Chest
5. Abdomen
6. Perineum/rectum
7. Extremities - fractures
8. Complete neurological examination
9. Appropriate roentgenograms, laboratory tests, and special studies.
10. "Tubes and fingers" in every orifice

D. Definitive Care

After identifying the patient's injuries, managing life-threatening problems, and obtaining special studies, definitive care begins. Definitive care, associated with the major trauma entities, is described in later chapters.

E. Transfer

If the patient's injuries exceed the institution's immediate treatment capabilities, the process of transferring the patient is initiated as soon as the need is identified. Delay in transferring the patient to a facility with a higher level of care may significantly increase the patient's risk of mortality.

Bibliography

1. American College of Surgeons: **Early Care of the Injured Patient.** Philadelphia, WB Saunders & Company, 1982.

2. American College of Surgeons: Technique of Helmet Removal from Injured Patients. **ACS Bulletin**, October,1980.

3. Collicott PE: Initial Assessment, in Mattox KL, Moore EE, Feliciano DV (ed),**Trauma**. Appleton-Lange, 1988.

4. McSwain NE Jr, Kerstein M (ed): **Evaluation and Management of Trauma**, Appleton-Century-Crofts, 1987.

5. McSwain NE Jr: Pneumatic Antishock Garment: State of the Art 1988. **Annals of Emergency Medicine**, May 1988; 17:506-525.

6. States JD, & Smith TG: Use of the Safety Belt Defense: The New York Experience American Association of Automotive Medicine Proceedings, October 1983; 27:77-85.

7. The Human Collision. Ontario Ministry of Transportation and Communication, September 1976.

8. Moore EE: Initial Resuscitation and Evaluation of the Injured Patient in Zuidema, GD, Rutherford, RB, Ballinger, WF. **The Management of Trauma**, WB Saunders & Company, 1985.

Skill Station I:
Initial Assessment

Chapter 1:
Initial
Assessment
and
Management

Skill
Station I

Equipment

1. Live patient model
2. Nurse assistant
3. Case scenarios with related roentgenograms
4. Blanket and sheet (or sufficient table padding for patient comfort)
5. Makeup and moulage
   a. Moulage piece: open femur fracture with blood adapter (optional)
   b. Makeup for bruises, abrasions, lacerations, and burns
   c. Artificial blood–various types
6. Items needed for each scenario:
   a. 4x4s, roller bandage, and tape
   b. Blood pressure cuff and stethoscope
   c. Penlite flashlight (optional)
   d. 1000 ml Ringer's lactate – two or three per patient
   e. Assorted intravenous catheters and needles, ie, #14-16-gauge over-the-needle catheter, #20-gauge Butterfly needle—two to four per patient
   f. Spine boards: long and short (optional)
   g. Semirigid cervical collar
   h. Oxygen masks
   i. Oral airway
   j. Leg traction splint; molded splints
   k. X-ray view box (optional)
   l. Laryngoscope blade, handle, and ET tube
   m. #5 tracheostomy tube for cricothyroidotomy
   n. #36 - 40 French chest tube and drainage collection device
   o. Scalpel handle
   p. Nasogastric tube
   q. Peritoneal lavage kit
   r. 12 ml and 50 ml syringes
   s. Indwelling urinary catheter and collection bag
   t. Bag-valve mask device and face mask (type that includes a one-way valve preventing back flow of air and secretions)
   u. Soft and rigid suction devices
   v. Portable electrocardiograph monitor (optional)
   w. Pneumatic antishock garment (optional)

Chapter 1:
Initial
Assessment
and
Management

Skill
Station I

Performance at this station will allow the participant to practice and demonstrate the following activities in a simulated clinical situation:

1. Using the four phases of patient assessment and management, verbalize to the instructor while systematically demonstrating the initial management required to stabilize each patient.

2. Using the primary survey assessment techniques, determine and demonstrate:

    a. Airway patency and cervical spine control.
    b. Breathing efficacy.
    c. Circulatory status with hemorrhage control.
    d. Disability: Neurological status.
    e. Exposure: Undress the patient.

3. Establish resuscitation (management) priorities in the multiply injured patient based upon findings from the primary survey.

4. Integrate appropriate history-taking as an invaluable aid in the assessment of the patient situation.

5. Identify the injury-producing mechanism and discuss the injuries that may exist and/or may be anticipated as a result of the mechanism of injury.

6. Using secondary survey techniques, assess the patient from head to toe.

7. Given a series of roentgenograms,

    a. Diagnose fractures.
    b. Differentiate associated injuries.

8. Outline the definitive care and management necessary to stabilize each patient in preparation for possible transport to a definitive-care facility.

Chapter 1:
Initial
Assessment
and
Management

Skill
Station I

Skills Procedures

Initial Assessment and Management

The history of a multiply injured patient will be presented to the participant. The participant is to demonstrate patient assessment and give directions for primary treatment and stabilization. Minimal resuscitation equipment, roentgenograms, and an assistant are available to the participant to **simulate** management procedures. The instructor will provide answers to the participant's questions, and physical findings. The participant should complete the patient survey in the sequence given.

Note: An evaluation listing **critical treatment decisions** for each patient situation is included in Section IV of the *ATLS Instructor Manual*. These evaluation forms and accompanying instructions will facilitate the faculty's evaluation of each student's performance.

I. Primary Survey and Resuscitation

The student should indicate the patient is to be undressed .

A. Airway Patency with Cervical Spine Control

1. Assessment

2. Management—establish a patent airway.

    a.   Chin lift or jaw thrust
    b.   Clear the airway of foreign bodies
    c.   Oropharyngeal airway
    d.   Orotracheal or nasotracheal intubation
    e.   Cricothyroidotomy

3. Maintain the cervical spine in aneutral position with manual immobilization as necessary when establishing an airway.

B. Breathing Control

1. Assessment

    a.   Expose the chest.
    b.   Determine the rate and depth of respirations.
    c.   Inspect and palpate for unilateral and bilateral chest movement, and any signs of injury.
    d.   Auscultate the chest bilaterally.

2. Management

    a.   Administer high concentrations of oxygen.
    b.   Alleviate tension pneumothorax.
    c.   Seal open pneumothorax.

**Chapter 1:
Initial
Assessment
and
Management**

**Skill
Station 1**

C.   Circulatory and Hemorrhage Control

1. Assessment

    a. Pulse.
        1) Quality
        2) Rate
        3) Regularity

    b. Color of skin
    c. Capillary blanch test
    d. Identify exsanguinating hemorrhage

2. Management

    a. Initiate two large-caliber intravenous catheters.
    b. Simultaneously obtain blood for hematologic and chemical analyses, type and crossmatch, and arterial blood gases.
    c. Initiate Ringer's lactate solution and blood replacement.
    d. Apply the pneumatic antishock garment as indicated or necessary.
    e. Apply direct pressure to bleeding site.
    f. Apply the pneumatic antishock garment or pneumatic splints to control hemorrhage.
    g. Attach the patient to an electrocardiographic monitor.
    h. Insert urinary and nasogastric catheters unless contraindicated.

D.   Disability–Brief Neurological Examination

1. Determine the level of consciousness using the AVPU method.

2. Assess the pupils for size, equality and reaction.

E.   Exposure

Completely undress the patient.

II. Secondary Survey and Management

A.   Head and Face

1. Assessment

    a. Inspection
    b. Palpation
    c. Re-evaluate pupils
    d. Cranial nerve function

2. Management

    a. Maintain airway
    b. Hemorrhage control

Chapter 1:
Initial
Assessment
and
Management

Skill
Station I

B. Neck

1. Assessment

    a. Inspection
    b. Palpation
    c. Auscultation
    d. Lateral, crosstable cervical spine roentgenogram.

2. Management

Maintain adequate inline immobilization of the cervical spine.

C. Chest

1. Assessment

    a. Inspection
    b. Auscultation
    c. Percussion
    d. Palpation

2. Management

    a. Pleural decompression
    b. Thoracentesis
    c. Pericardiocentesis
    d. Chest roentgenogram

D. Abdomen

1. Assessment

    a. Inspection
    b. Auscultation
    c. Percussion
    d. Palpation

2. Management

    a. Peritoneal lavage, if indicated
    b. Application of pneumatic antishock garment, if indicated

E. Perineal and Rectal Exam

Evaluate for

1. Anal sphincter tone

2. Rectal blood

3. Bowel wall integrity

4. Prostate position

5. Blood at the urinary meatus

**Chapter 1:
Initial
Assessment
and
Management**

**Skill
Station 1**

6. Scrotal hematoma

F. Back

Evaluate for:

1. Bony deformity

2. Evidence of penetrating or blunt trauma

G. Extremities

1. Assessment

   a. Inspection: Deformity, expanding hematoma
   b. Palpation: Tenderness, crepitation, abnormal movement

2. Management

   a. Appropriate splinting for fractures
   b. Use of pneumatic antishock garment
   c. Relief of pain
   d. Tetanus immunization

H. Neurologic

1. Assessment

   a. Sensorimotor evaluation
   b. Paralysis
   c. Paresis

2. Management

Adequate immobilization of entire patient

IV. Stabilization and Transport

Outline rationale for patient transfer, transfer procedures, and patient's needs during transfer.

Chapter 2:
Airway Management and
Ventilation

Objectives:

Upon completion of this topic, the physician will be able to explain and demonstrate the principles of airway management.

Specifically, the physician will be able to:

A. Recognize those conditions associated with airway and ventilatory compromise in the acutely injured as well as the stabilized trauma victim.

B. Discuss the principles of airway intervention and ventilatory management.

C. Demonstrate basic and advanced methods of airway intervention.

D. Perform transtracheal insufflation and surgical cricothyroidotomy during the surgical practicum.

E. Demonstrate one-man and two-man techniques for ventilating a patient.

**Chapter 2:
Airway
Management
and
Ventilation**

I. Introduction

The upper and lower airway are of concern in **any** patient sustaining multiple trauma, because injury to either the upper or lower airway can compromise ventilation. Therefore, both areas require attention. An airway must be secured, oxygen delivered via a face mask with a reservoir device, and ventilatory support provided. **Supplemental oxygen must be administered to all trauma patients.**

Early preventable deaths from airway problems after trauma are frequently due to:

1. The multiplicity of signs and symptoms, which may overwhelm the physician's senses and delay airway management.

2. Failure to recognize subtle or even obvious indicators for airway intervention in patients with airway and ventilatory compromise.

3. Faulty judgment in selecting the correct airway maneuver.

4. Limited experience with airway skill provision.

II. Airway and Ventilatory Compromise

A. Awareness

Airway compromise may be acute, insidious, progressive, and recurrent. Altered consciousness represents the single most frequent indication to provide an airway with endotracheal intubation. The unconscious, head-injured patient, the patient obtunded from alcohol and/or drugs, and the patient with thoracic injuries may have compromised ventilatory effort. In these patients, endotracheal intubation is intended to: 1) provide an airway, 2) deliver supplementary oxygen, and 3) support ventilation. **Preventing hypercarbia is critical in managing the trauma patient, especially if the patient has sustained a head injury.** (See Chapter 6–Head Trauma.)

Trauma to the face and/or neck, with actual compromise to the airway lumen, is another indication for airway intervention. The mechanism for this injury is exemplified by the unbelted passenger/driver who is thrown into the windshield and dash. Trauma to the midface may produce fractures-dislocations with compromise to the nasal and oral pharynx. Fractures of the mandible may result in the loss of normal mastication muscle support and subsequent obstruction of the hypopharynx by the tongue. Facial fractures may be associated with hemorrhage and increased secretions, causing additional airway compromise. Injuries to the neck may affect the airway as a result of direct trauma to the larynx, the supporting structures of the airway (mandible), or hemorrhage with secondary compression.

B. Recognition

The most important question one can ask the trauma patient is, "How are you?" Failure to respond implies an altered level of consciousness. A positive, appropriate **verbal** response indicates that the airway is patent, ventilation intact, and brain perfusion adequate. Any inappropriate response may suggest airway/ventilatory compromise.

1. **Look** to see if the patient is agitated or obtunded. Agitation suggests hypoxia, and obtundation suggests hypercarbia. Cyanosis indicates hypoxemia due to inadequate ventilation. **Remember,** patients who refuse to lie down quietly may be attempting to clear their secretions by sitting up.

2. **Listen** for abnormal sounds. Snoring, gurgling, and gargling sounds may be associated with partial occlusion of the pharynx. Hoarseness (dysphonia) implies laryngeal obstruction. The abusive/abrasive patient may be hypoxic and should not be presumed intoxicated.

3. **Feel** for the movement of air with the expiratory effort and quickly determine if the trachea is midline.

III. Management

Management objectives for airway compromise include: 1) securing an intact airway, 2) protecting the jeopardized airway, and 3) providing an airway if none is available. Basic, advanced, and surgical airway intervention techniques must be applied with the full realization that the patient may have a cervical spine injury. The neck must be securely immobilized until the possibility of a spinal injury has been ruled out with suitable roentgenographic studies, or the injury has been recognized and appropriately managed. A patient wearing a helmet is no exception. If a cervical spine injury is present, the helmet should be removed appropriately and safely.

A. Basic Life Support

For the patient with an altered sensorium, the tongue prolapses backward and obstructs the hypopharynx. This simple obstruction can be readily corrected by the chin-lift or jaw-thrust maneuver. The airway can then be maintained with an oral or pharyngeal airway.

1. Chin lift

The fingers of one hand are placed under the mandible, which is gently lifted upward to bring the chin anterior. The thumb of the same hand lightly depresses the lower lip to open the mouth. The thumb may also be placed behind the lower incisors and, simultaneously, the chin gently lifted. The chin-lift maneuver **should not hyperextend the neck.** The chin lift is the method of choice for the trauma victim because it does not risk compromising a possible cervical spine fracture, or converting a fracture without cord injury into one with cord injury.

2. Jaw thrust

The jaw-thrust maneuver is performed by grasping the angles of the lower jaw, one hand on each side, and displacing the mandible forward. When this method is used with the mouth-to-face mask (using the type of equipment that prevents backward flow of air and secretions), a good seal and adequate ventilation are achieved.

3. Suction

Blood and secretions should be removed with a rigid suction device (tonsil suction tip). Patients with facial injuries may have associated cribriform plate fractures, and the routine use of the soft suction catheter or the nasogastric tube inserted through the nose may be complicated by passage of the tubes into the cranial vault.

4. Oropharyngeal airway

The oral airway is inserted into the mouth behind the tongue. This technique is facilitated by using a tongue blade to depress the tongue and then inserting the airway posteriorly. The airway must not push the tongue backward and block, rather than clear, the airway.

An alternative technique is to insert the oral airway upside-down, so its concavity is directed upward, until the soft palate is encountered. At this point, the airway is rotated 180 degrees, the concavity is directed caudad, and the airway is slipped into place over the tongue. This method should not be used for children, because the rotation of the airway may damage the teeth.

5. Nasopharyngeal airway

The nasal airway is simply inserted into one nostril to provide adequate passage into the hypopharynx. The nasal airway may be inferior to the oral airway, but unlike the oral airway, the responsive patient tolerates it well. It should be lubricated, then inserted into the nostril that appears to be unobstructed. If obstruction is encountered during introduction of the airway, stop and try the other nostril.

B. Advanced Airway Intervention

The urgency of the situation and the circumstances surrounding the need for airway intervention often dictate the specific route and method to be used. Oral and nasal endotracheal intubation are the methods used most frequently. The potential for concomitant cervical spine injury is of major concern in the patient requiring an airway. The algorithm that appears at the conclusion of this chapter exemplifies a scheme by which the decision for the appropriate route of airway management can be made.

1. Endotracheal intubation

For the unconscious patient who has sustained blunt trauma and needs an airway, first determine the urgency for that airway. If there is no immediate need, then a roentgenogram of the cervical spine should be obtained. A normal lateral cervical spine roentgenograph is reassuring and allows safe oroendotracheal intubation with midline immobilization of the head and neck. However, a normal lateral cervical spine film does **not** rule out a cervical spine injury. Spinal immobilization should be maintained until removed by the neurosurgical or orthopedic consultant. If no cervical spine fractures are noted, **oral endotracheal intubation** should be performed. If a fracture is seen or suspected, **nasoendotracheal intubation** may be performed according to clinical judgment.

If the immediate need for an airway **precludes radiographic evaluation of the cervical spine**, and if the patient is breathing, **nasoendotracheal intubation** should be attempted. If the patient is **apneic,** orotracheal intubation with inline manual cervical immobilization should be attempted.

Malpositioning of the endotracheal tube must be considered in all patients who arrive at the hospital with an endotracheal tube presumably positioned properly. The tube may have been inserted into a mainstem bronchus, or dislodged during patient transport from the field or another hospital. Placement can be checked quickly by listening for equal breath sounds bilaterally, and listening over the stomach to determine unintentional esophageal intubation.

If the patient's condition permits, fiberoptic endoscopy may facilitate difficult oral or nasoendotracheal intubation. The endoscopic techniques may be used for selected cases of maxillofacial and cervical spine injury, and for stocky patients with short necks. If these injuries or conditions preclude oral or nasal endotracheal intubation, the physician may proceed directly to surgical techniques: needle or surgical cricothyroidotomy.

The esophageal obturator airway is an ineffective device with which to establish an airway. However, physicians may encounter patients in whom an esophageal obturator airway (EOA or EGTA) has been inserted. If an unconscious patient has an EOA or EGTA in place, the patient must be endotracheally intubated before removing it. Replacement with an endotracheal tube is not necessary if the patient regains consciousness. In fact, suction should be obtained, the head turned to the side if a neck injury has been excluded, the cuff deflated, and the EOA removed.

C. Surgical Airway Intervention

Inability to intubate the trachea is the only indication for creating a surgical airway.

When edema of the glottis, fracture of the larynx, or severe oropharyngeal hemorrhage obstructs the airway and an endotracheal tube **cannot** be placed through the cords, a surgical cricothyroidotomy may be performed to allow air passage. Insertion of a needle through the cricothyroid membrane or into the trachea is an acceptable alternative to a surgical cricothyroidotomy. An emergency tracheostomy, done under emergency conditions, is difficult to perform, is often associated with profuse bleeding, and may require too much time to perform.

1. Jet insufflation of the airway

Needle cricothyroidotomy is an acceptable alternative method to the surgical route and is preferable in an emergency situation for a child under the age of 12 years.

Use of the jet insufflation technique can provide up to 45 minutes of extra time so that intubation can be accomplished on an urgent rather than an emergent basis.

The jet insufflation technique is performed by placing a large-caliber plastic cannula, #12- to #14-gauge, in the trachea below the level of the obstruction. The cannula is then connected to wall oxygen at 15 liters/minute (40 to 50 PSI) with either a Y-connector or a side hole cut in the tubing attached between the oxygen source and the plastic cannula. Intermittent ventilation, one second on and four seconds off, can then be achieved by placing the thumb over the open end of the Y-connector or the side hole. The patient can be adequately ventilated for **only** 30 to 45 minutes using this technique. During the four seconds that the oxygen is not being delivered under pressure, some exhalation will occur. Because of this inadequate exhalation, carbon dioxide may accumulate and limit the use of this technique.

Jet insufflation may also be used for foreign body obstruction in the glottic area. Not only can ventilation and oxygenation be performed, but the high pressure may expel the impacted material into the hypopharynx, where it can be readily removed.

2. Surgical cricothyroidotomy

Surgical cricothyroidotomy is easily performed by making a skin incision that extends through the cricothyroid membrane. A curved hemostat may be inserted to dilate the opening and a small endotracheal tube or tracheostomy tube (preferably 5 mm to 7 mm) can be inserted. When the endotracheal tube is used, the cervical collar can be reapplied. One must be alert to the possibility that the endotracheal tube can become malpositioned. Should long-term tracheal intubation be required, the cricothyroidotomy can be replaced with a tracheostomy. Care must be taken, especially with children, to avoid damage to the cricoid cartilage, which is the only circumferential support to the upper trachea. Therefore, surgical cricothyroidotomy is not recommended for children under 12 years. (See Chapter 10—Pediatric Trauma.)

D. Oxygenation and Ventilation

The primary goal of ventilation is to achieve maximum cellular oxygenation which is promoted in the trauma patient by providing an environment rich in oxygen (using high-flow oxygen at 10 to 12 liters/minute and a tight-fitting mask), and sustained gas exchange at the alveolar capillary membrane through improved ventilatory efforts.

1. Oxygenation

High-flow oxygen delivery via a nasal cannula or simple plastic face mask fails to provide an FIO_2 of at least 0.85, and therefore should not be used for the trauma patient. However, a tight-fitting, oxygen reservoir face mask with high-flow oxygen delivery can deliver an FIO_2 of 0.85.

2. Ventilation

The hypoxic and/or apneic patient must be ventilated and oxygenated before intubation is attempted.

Ventilation can be achieved by mouth-to-face mask (using the type of equipment that prevents backward flow of air and secretions), or bag-valve-face-mask. **Frequently, only one person is present to provide ventilation; under these circumstances, mouth-to-face mask ventilation is the preferred method. Studies suggest that one-person ventilation techniques, using a bag-valve mask, are less effective** than two-person techniques in which both hands can be used to assure a good seal.

Intubation of the hypoventilated and/or apneic patient may not be successful initially and may require multiple attempts. Prolonged efforts to intubate without intermittent ventilation **must** be avoided. The physician should practice taking a deep breath when intubation is first attempted. When the physician must breathe, the attempted intubation should be aborted, and the patient ventilated.

With intubation of the trachea accomplished, assisted ventilation should follow, using positive-pressure breathing techniques. A volume- or pressure-regulated respirator can be employed, depending on availability of equipment. The physician should be alert for the complications secondary to changes in intrathoracic pressure, which can convert a simple pneumothorax to a tension pneumothorax, or even create a pneumothorax secondary to barotrauma.

IV. Summary

A. An altered level of consciousness is the most common cause of upper airway obstruction.

B. Beware of a cervical spine injury during airway management.

C. The chin lift is the preferred manual method to open the airway.

D. Oral and nasopharyngeal airways maintain a patent airway.

E. If a cervical spine injury is radiologically absent, oral intubation may be performed.

F. When a cervical spine injury is certain or suspected, nasotracheal intubation should be performed.

G. Beware of malpositioning of the endotracheal tube.

H. Inability to intubate requires the utilization of surgical airway techniques.

I. Intermittent ventilation between attempts at intubation and postintubation ventilation are vital concerns.

Indications for Intubation and Surgical Airway

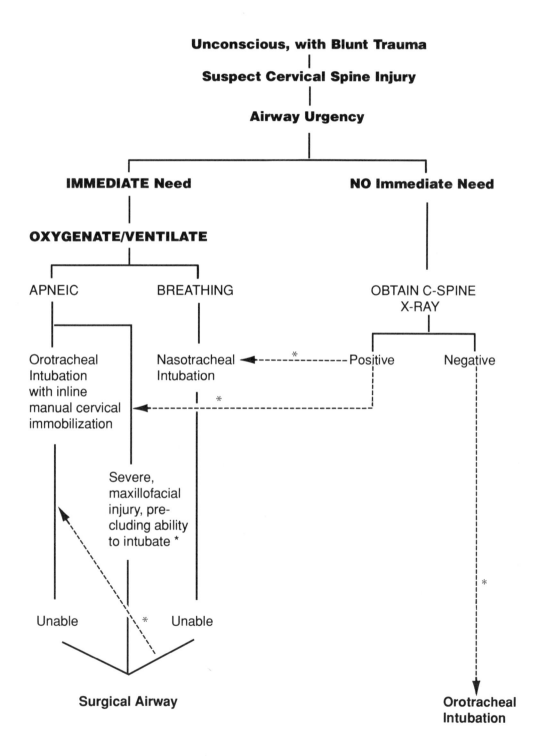

Unconscious, with Blunt Trauma

Suspect Cervical Spine Injury

Airway Urgency

IMMEDIATE Need

NO Immediate Need

OXYGENATE/VENTILATE

APNEIC   BREATHING   OBTAIN C-SPINE X-RAY

Orotracheal Intubation with inline manual cervical immobilization

Nasotracheal Intubation ◄--------- * --------- Positive   Negative

Severe, maxillofacial injury, precluding ability to intubate *

Unable   *   Unable

Surgical Airway

Orotracheal Intubation

* Proceed according to clinical judgment

Bibliography

1. Aprahamian C, Thompson BM, Finger WA et al: Experimental Cervical Spine Injury Model: Evaluation of Airway Management and Splinting Techniques. **Annals of Emergency Medicine** 1984;13(8):584-587.

2. Attia RR, Battit GE, and Murphy JD: Transtracheal Ventilation. **Journal of the American Medical Association** 1975; 234:1152-1153.

3. Brantigan CO and Grow JB: Cricothyroidotomy: Elective Use of Respiratory Problems Requiring Tracheotomy. **The Journal of Thoracic and Cardiovascular Surgery** 1976;71:72-81.

4. Bouzarth WR: Editorial: Intracranial Nasogastric Tube Insertion. **Journal of Trauma** 1978;18:819.

5. Butler RM and Moser FH: The Padded Dash Syndrome: Blunt Trauma to the Larynx and Trachea. **Laryngoscope** 1968; 78:1172-1182.

6. Emergency Percutaneous and Transtracheal Ventilation. **Journal of American College of Emergency Physicians/Annals of Emergency Medicine**; October 1979; 8(10):396.

7. Iserson KV: Blind Nasotracheal Intubation. **Annals of Emergency Medicine** 1981;10:468.

8. Fremstad JD, and Martin SH: Lethal Complication from Insertion of Nasogastric Tube after Severe Basilar Skull Fracture. **Journal of Trauma** 1978;18:820-822.

9. Greenbaum DM, Poggi J, and Grace WJ: Esophageal Obstruction During Oxygen Administration: A New Method for Use in Resuscitation. **Chest** 1974;65:188-191.

10. Greene R, and Stark P: Trauma of the Larynx and Trachea. **Radiologic Clinics of North America** 1978;16:309-320.

11. Guildner CW: Resuscitation–Opening the Airway. A Comparative Study of Techniques for Opening an Airway Obstructed by the Tongue. **Journal of American College of Emergency Physicians** 1976;5:588-590.

12. Johnson KR, Genovesi MG, Lassar KH: Esophageal Obturator Airway: Use and Complications. **Journal of American College of Emergency Physicians** 1976;5:36-39.

13. Kress TD, et al: Cricothyroidotomy. **Annals of Emergency Medicine** 1982; 11:197.

14. Manoranijan CS, Jesudian MD, Harrison BA, et al: Bag-valve- mask ventilation; two rescuers are better than one: Preliminary report. **Critical Care Medicine** 1985;13(2) pp 122-123.

15. Nahum AM: Immediate Care of Acute Blunt Laryngeal Trauma. **Journal of Trauma** 1969; 9:112-125.

16. Nasotracheal Intubation in the Emergency Department. **Critical Care Medicine** 1980; 8:667-82.

17. Rogers LF: Injuries Peculiar to Traffic Accidents: Seat Belt Syndrome, Laryngeal Fracture, Hangman's Fracture. **Texas Medicine** 1974; 70-77-83.

18. Seshul MB Sr, Sinn DP, and Gerlock AJ Jr: The Andy Gump Fracture of the Mandible: A Cause of Respiratory Obstruction or Distress. **Journal of Trauma** 1978; 18:611-612.

19. Strate R, and Fischer RP: Midesophageal Perforations by Esophageal Obturator Airways. **Journal of Trauma** 1976; 16:503-509.

20. Tintinalli J et al: Complications of Nasotracheal Intubation. **Annals of Emergency Medicine** March 1981; 10:142- 44.

**Chapter 2:
Airway
Management
and
Ventilation**

Skill Station II: Airway Management

Chapter 2:
Airway
Management
and
Ventilation

Skill
Station II

Equipment

1. Adult intubation manikins–two or three
2. Infant intubation manikin–one or two
3. Adult oroendotracheal tubes–assorted sizes
4. Adult nasoendotracheal tubes–assorted sizes
5. Infant endotracheal tubes–assorted sizes, uncuffed
6. Laryngoscope handles–three or four
7. Laryngoscope blades–infant and adult sizes, straight and curved
8. Extra batteries for laryngoscope handles
9. Extra laryngoscope bulbs
10. Stethoscopes–two
11. Lubricant (ie, silicone spray that accompanies intubation manikin)
12. Nasal anesthetic spray (simulation purposes only)
13. Semirigid cervical collar (applied to one adult intubation manikin)
14. Magill forcep–one
15. Malleable endotracheal tube stylet–two or three
16. Oropharyngeal airway–assorted sizes
17. Nasopharyngeal airway–assorted sizes
18. Bag-valve mask device–one or two
19. Pocket face mask–one or two (**Note:** type that includes a one-way valve preventing the back flow of air and secretions)
20. Rigid suction device–one (tonsil suction device)

Objectives

Performance at this station will allow the participant to practice and demonstrate the following skills on adult and infant intubation manikins.

1. Ventilate the patient, comparing ventilatory volumes delivered via the rescuer's lungs and a face mask versus the bag-valve-mask device.

2. Insert oral and nasal pharyngeal airways.

3. Using both oral and nasal routes, intubate the trachea of an adult intubation manikin, within the guidelines listed, and provide effective ventilation.

4. Intubate the trachea of an infant intubation manikin with an endotracheal tube within the guidelines listed, and provide effective ventilation.

5. Relate the indications and complications of trauma to airway management when performing oral endotracheal intubation and nasotracheal intubation.

Chapter 2:
Airway
Management
and
Ventilation

Skill
Station II

Five procedures for acute airway management are outlined in Skill Station II: **Procedures**

1. Oropharyngeal airway insertion

2. Nasopharyngeal airway insertion

3. Ventilation without Intubation

4. Orotracheal intubation

5. Nasotracheal intubation

6. Infant endotracheal intubation

Skills Procedures

Airway Management

Chapter 2:
Airway
Management
and
Ventilation

Skill
Station II

I. Oropharyngeal Airway Insertion

A. Select the proper-sized airway. (Place the airway against the patient's face. The correctly sized airway will extend from the center of the patient's mouth to the angle of the jaw.)

B. Open the patient's mouth with either the chin lift maneuver or the crossed-finger technique (scissors technique).

C. Insert the tip of the airway, in an upside-down position, into the patient's mouth so the concavity of the airway is directed upward.

D. Gently slide the airway along the roof of the mouth to the soft palate.

E. Gently rotate the airway 180 degrees, direct the concavity of the airway caudad, and slip the airway over the tongue.

F. Ventilate the patient with a pocket face mask or bag-valve-mask device.

II. Nasopharyngeal Airway Insertion

A. Assess the nasal passages for any apparent obstruction (polyps, fractures, hemorrhage, etc).

B. Select the appropriately sized airway.

C. Lubricate the nasal pharyngeal airway with a water-soluble lubricant or tap water.

D. Insert the tip of the airway into the nostril and direct it posteriorly and towards the ear.

E. Gently pass the nasal pharyngeal airway through the nostril into the hypopharynx with a slight rotating motion, until the flange rests against the nostril.

F. Ventilate the patient with a pocket face mask or bag- valve-mask device.

III. Ventilation Without Intubation

A. Mouth-to-Pocket Face Mask (One-Person Technique)

1. Attach oxygen tubing to the face mask. Oxygen flow rate should be 12 L/minute.

2. Apply the face mask to the patient, using both hands.

**Chapter 2:
Airway
Management
and
Ventilation**

**Skill
Station II**

3. Assure an adequate seal of the mask to the face.

4. Secure an open airway by using the jaw-thrust or chin-lift maneuver.

5. Taking a deep breath, place your mouth over the mouth port and blow.

6. Assess the ventilatory efforts by observing the patient's chest movement.

7. Ventilate the patient in this manner every five seconds.

B. Bag-Valve-Mask Ventilation (Two-person Technique)

1. Select the appropriately sized mask to fit the patient's face.

2. Connect the oxygen tubing to the bag-valve device, and adjust the flow of oxygen to 12 L/minute.

3. Assure that the patient's airway is patent and secured by previously described techniques.

4. The **first person** applies the mask to the patient's face, ascertaining a tight seal with both hands.

5. The **second person** ventilates the patient by squeezing the bag with both hands.

6. The adequacy of ventilation is assessed by observing the patient's chest movement.

7. The patient should be ventilated in this manner every five seconds.

III. Adult Orotracheal Intubation

Note: This procedure is usually used on patients for whom a cervical spine injury has been ruled out radiologically.

A. Assure that adequate ventilation and oxygenation are in progress.

B. Connect laryngoscope blade and handle; check the bulb for brightness.

C. Have an assistant manually immobilize the head and neck.

D. Hold the laryngoscope in the left hand.

E. Insert the laryngoscope into the right side of the patient's mouth, displacing the tongue to the left.

F. Visually examine the epiglottis and then the vocal cords.

G. Gently insert the endotracheal tube into the trachea without applying pressure on the teeth or oral tissues.

H. Inflate the cuff with enough air to provide an adequate seal. **Do not overinflate the cuff.**

I. Check the placement of the endotracheal tube by bag-valve-to-tube ventilation.

**Chapter 2:
Airway
Management
and
Ventilation**

**Skill
Station II**

J. Visually observe lung expansion with ventilation.

K. Auscultate the chest and abdomen with a stethoscope to ascertain tube position.

L. If endotracheal intubation is not accomplished within seconds or in the same time required to hold your breath before exhaling, discontinue attempts, ventilate the patient with a bag-valve-mask device, and try again.

M. Obtain a chest film to ascertain exact placement of the endotracheal tube.

Complications of Orotracheal Intubation

1. Esophageal intubation, leading to hypoxia and death.

2. Right mainstem bronchus intubation, resulting in collapse of the left lung and pneumothorax.

3. Inability to intubate, leading to hypoxia and death.

4. Induction of vomiting, leading to aspiration, hypoxia, and death.

5. Dislocation of the mandible.

6. Fracture of the epiglottis.

7. Airway hemorrhage secondary to trauma.

8. Avulsion tear of the vocal cords (usually from the stylet).

9. Chipping or loosening of the teeth (caused by levering of the laryngoscope blade against the teeth).

10. Rupture/leak of the endotracheal tube cuff, resulting in loss of seal during ventilation, and necessitating reintubation.

11. Dislocation of the cervical spine during hyperextension or hyperflexion.

12. Neck strain during hyperextension.

13. Atlanto-occipital dislocation.

14. Potential fracture of anterior cervical spine fusion.

15. Conversion of cervical spine injury without neurological deficit to cervical spine injury with neurological deficit.

IV. Adult Nasotracheal Intubation

Note: This procedure is usually performed on patients for whom a cervical spine injury exists or cannot be ruled out by prior roentgenograms due to life-threatening conditions.

A. If a cervical spine fracture is suspected, leave the cervical collar in place to assist in maintaining immobilization of the neck.

**Chapter 2:
Airway
Management
and
Ventilation**

**Skill
Station II**

B. Assure that adequate ventilation and oxygenation are in progress.

C. If the patient is **conscious**, spray the nasal passage with an anesthetic and vasoconstrictor to anesthetize and constrict the mucosa. If the patient is **unconscious**, it is adequate to spray the nasal passage only with a vasoconstrictor.

D. Have an assistant maintain manual immobilization of the head and neck.

E. Lubricate the nasal endotracheal tube, with a local anesthetic jelly and insert the tube (with or without a stylet) into the nostril.

F. Guide the tube slowly but firmly into the nasal passage, going up from the nostril (to avoid the large inferior turbinate) and then backward and down into the nasopharynx. The curve of the tube should be aligned to facilitate passage along this curved course.

G. As the tube passes through the nose and into the nasopharynx, it must turn downward to pass through the pharynx.

H. Once the tube has entered the pharynx, listen to the airflow emanating from the endotracheal tube. Advance the tube until the sound of the moving air is maximal, suggesting location of the tip at the opening of the trachea. While listening to air movement, determine the point of inhalation and advance the tube quickly. If tube placement is unsuccessful, repeat the procedure by applying gentle pressure on the thyroid cartilage. If the procedure is still unsuccessful, the thyroid cartilage can be directed cephalad to facilitate tube placement. **Remember, intermittently ventilate and oxygenate the patient.**

I. Optional method: If an endotracheal stylet is utilized, bend the lower end of the tube (approximately the last one-fourth) to a near 90-degree angle. As the tube is inserted, the end of the tube should point to the ipsilateral ear. Be sure that the stylet is recessed one-half inch from the end of the tube to prevent trauma during insertion. As the tube is gently but firmly guided into the pharynx, apply the chin lift maneuver and depress the tongue with your thumb to facilitate entrance of the tube through the glottis and vocal cords. Continue to advance the tube with gentle pressure as you withdraw the stylet.

J. Inflate the cuff with enough air to provide an adequate seal. Avoid overinflation.

K. Check the placement of the endotracheal tube by bag-valve-to-tube ventilation.

L. Visually observe lung expansion with ventilation.

M. Auscultate the chest and abdomen with a stethoscope to ascertain tube position.

N. If endotracheal intubation is not accomplished within 30 seconds, discontinue attempts, ventilate the patient with a bag-valve-mask device, and try again.

O. Obtain a chest film to ascertain exact placement of the endotracheal tube.

Complications of Nasotracheal Intubation

1. Esophageal intubation, leading to hypoxia and death.

2. Induction of vomiting and aspiration.

3. Trauma to the airway resulting in hemorrhage and potential aspiration.

4. Insertion of the tube past the carina into the right mainstem bronchus resulting in ventilation of the right lung only.

5. Trauma to the vocal cords.

V. Infant Orotracheal Intubation

A. Ensure that adequate ventilation and oxygenation are in progress.

B. Connect the laryngoscope blade and handle; check the light bulb for brilliance.

C. Hold the laryngoscope in the left hand.

D. Insert the laryngoscope blade in the right side of the mouth, moving the tongue to the left.

E. Observe the epiglottis, then the vocal cords.

F. Insert the endotracheal tube.

G. Check the placement of the tube by bag-valve-to-tube ventilation.

H. Check the placement of the endotracheal tube by observing lung inflations and auscultating of the chest with a stethoscope.

I. Obtain a chest film to ascertain exact placement of the endotracheal tube.

Chapter 2:
Airway
Management
and
Ventilation

Skill
Station II

**Chapter 2:
Airway
Management
and
Ventilation**

**Skill
Station II**

American College of Surgeons

Skill Station III: Cricothyroidotomy

**Chapter 2:
Airway
Management
and
Ventilation**

**Skill
Station III**

This surgical procedure, if performed on a live, anesthetized animal, must be conducted in a USDA–Registered Animal Laboratory Facility. (See *Instructor Manual*, Section II, Chapter 10–Animal Laboratory Guidelines and Protocols.)

Equipment

1. Live, anesthetized animals
2. Licensed veterinarian (see reference to guidelines above)
3. Animal trough, ropes (sandbags optional)
4. Electric shears with #40 blade
5. Animal intubation equipment
   a. Endotracheal tubes
   b. Laryngoscope blade and handle
   c. Respirator with 15-mm adapter
6. Tables or instrument stands
7. #12- to #14-gauge over-the-needle catheters (8.5 cm in length)
8. Antiseptic swabs
9. Pediatric (3.0 mm) endotracheal tube adapter
10. Jet insufflation equipment
    a. Y-connector and oxygen tubing
    b. Wall-mounted oxygen device or oxygen tank with flow meter
11. 6-ml and 10-ml syringes
12. Surgical instruments
    a. Scalpel handles with #10 and #11 blades
    b. Hemostats
    c. Tracheal hook (optional)
    d. Tracheal spreader (optional)
    e. Small rake retractors
13. Cricothyroidotomy tubes or #5 tracheostomy tubes
14. Twill-tape
15. 4x4 sponges
16. Surgical garb (gloves, shoe covers, and scrub suits or cover gowns)

Chapter 2:
Airway
Management
and
Ventilation

Skill
Station III

1. Performance at this station will allow the participant to practice and demonstrate the technique of needle cricothyroidotomy and surgical cricothyroidotomy on a live, anesthetized animal.

2. Upon completion of this station, the participant will be able to identify the surface markings and structures to be noted while performing a needle cricothyroidotomy and surgical cricothyroidotomy.

3. Upon completion of this station, the participant will be able to discuss the indications of needle cricothyroidotomy and surgical cricothyroidotomy.

4. Upon completion of this station, the participant will be able to discuss complications of these procedures.

Objectives

1. Needle Cricothyroidotomy

2. Surgical Cricothyroidotomy

Procedures

Skills Procedures
Cricothyroidotomy

Chapter 2:
Airway
Management
and
Ventilation

Skill
Station III

I. Needle Cricothyroidotomy

A. Place the patient in a supine position.

B. Palpate the cricothyroid membrane, anteriorly, between the thyroid cartilage and cricoid cartilage.

C. Surgically prep the area, using antiseptic swabs.

D. Assemble a #12- or #14-gauge, 8.5 cm, over-the-needle catheter to a 6- to 12-ml syringe.

E. Puncture the skin midline and directly over the cricothyroid membrane (ie, midsagittal).

F. Direct the needle at a 45-degree angle caudally.

G. Carefully insert the needle through the lower half of the cricothyroid membrane, aspirating as the needle is advanced.

H. Aspiration of air signifies entry into the tracheal lumen.

I. Withdraw the stylet while gently advancing the catheter downward into position, being careful not to perforate the posterior wall of the trachea.

J. Attach the catheter needle hub to a 3.0-mm pediatric endotracheal tube adapter.

K. Then, connect this "cricothyroidotomy" adapter to oxygen tubing with a Y-connector. The oxygen flow meter should be set at 15 L/minute (50 PSI). **Note:** Adequate PaO_2 can be maintained for only 30 to 45 minutes.

Intermittent ventilation can be achieved by placing the thumb over the open end of the Y-connector, using the rhythm of one second on and four seconds off.

L. Observe lung inflations and auscultate the chest for adequate ventilation.

M. Secure the apparatus to the patient's neck.

Complications of Needle Cricothyroidotomy

1. Asphyxia
2. Aspiration
3. Cellulitis
4. Esophageal perforation
5. Exsanguinating hematoma
6. Hematoma
7. Posterior tracheal wall perforation

**Chapter 2:
Airway
Management
and
Ventilation**

**Skill
Station III**

8. Subcutaneous and/or mediastinal emphysema
9. Thyroid perforation
10. Inadequate ventilations leading to hypoxia and death

II. Surgical Cricothyroidotomy

A. Place the patient in a supine position with the neck in a neutral position. Palpate the thyroid notch, cricothyroid interval, and the sternal notch for orientation.

B. Surgically prep and anesthetize the area locally, if the patient is conscious.

C. Stabilize the thyroid cartilage with the left hand.

D. Make a skin incision over the lower one-half of the cricothyroid membrane. Carefully incise through the membrane.

E. Insert the scalpel handle into the incision and rotate it 90 degrees to open the airway. (A tracheal spreader may be used instead of the scalpel handle.)

F. Insert an appropriately sized, cuffed endotracheal tube or tracheostomy tube into the cricothyroid membrane incision, directing the tube distally into the trachea.

G. Inflate the cuff and ventilate the patient.

H. Observe lung inflations and auscultate the chest for adequate ventilation.

I. Secure the endotracheal or tracheostomy tube to the patient to prevent dislodging.

J. Caution: Do not cut or remove the cricothyroid cartilage.

Complications of Surgical Cricothyroidotomy

1. Asphyxia
2. Aspiration (eg, blood)
3. Cellulitis
4. Creation of a false passage into the tissues
5. Subglottic stenosis/edema
6. Laryngeal stenosis
7. Hemorrhage or hematoma formation
8. Laceration of the esophagus
9. Laceration of the trachea
10. Mediastinal emphysema
11. Vocal cord paralysis, hoarseness

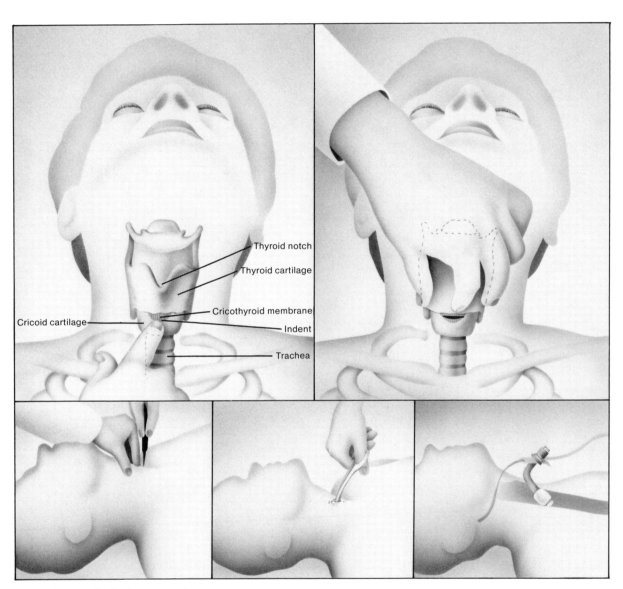

Thyroid notch
Thyroid cartilage
Cricothyroid membrane
Cricoid cartilage
Indent
Trachea

Surgical Cricothyroidotomy

**Chapter 2:
Airway
Management
and
Ventilation**

**Skill
Station III**

Chapter 3:
Shock

Objectives:

Upon completion of this topic, the physician will be able to identify and apply principles of management related to the initial diagnosis and treatment of shock in the injured patient. Specifically, the physician will be able to:

A. Define shock.

B. Identify the basic clinical shock syndrome and correlate the patient's acute clinical signs with the degree of volume deficit.

C. Discuss the basic principles that apply to the emergency treatment of hemorrhagic shock and their application to the patient's clinical response to therapy.

D. Discuss the clinical significance of fluid management for problems unique to the trauma patient.

E. Demonstrate various techniques of central and peripheral intravenous line insertion, including cutdowns.

F. Discuss the indications, contraindications, and dangers of inhospital use of the pneumatic antishock garment.

Chapter 3:
Shock

I. Introduction

The **initial step** in managing shock in the injured patient is to **recognize its presence**. No laboratory tests immediately diagnose shock. The initial diagnosis is based on clinical appreciation of the presence of inadequate organ perfusion. Thus the definition of shock as an abnormality of the circulatory system that results in **inadequate organ perfusion**, also becomes an operative tool for diagnosis and treatment.

The **second step** in the initial management of shock is to **identify the probable cause of the shock state.** For the trauma patient this identification process is directly related to the mechanism of injury. All types of shock may be present in the trauma patient. The majority of injured patients in shock are hypovolemic, but cardiogenic shock may be the cause and must be considered in patients with specific injuries above the diaphragm. The clinical situations that make this problem more likely will be discussed later in this chapter. Neurogenic shock results from extensive injury to the central nervous system or the spinal cord. **For all practical purposes, shock does not result from isolated head injuries.** Septic shock is unusual but must be considered for patients whose arrival at the emergency facility has been greatly delayed.

The end result of inadequately treated hypoperfusion is organ failure leading to immediate or delayed patient demise. For that reason, **the treatment of shock is directed toward restoring cellular and organ perfusion with adequately oxygenated blood,** rather than merely restoring the patient's blood pressure and pulse rate. Therefore, **vasopressors are contraindicated** for the treatment of hemorrhagic shock.

A significant percentage of injured patients who are in hypovolemic shock will require surgical intervention, and many of these will require early intervention to relieve the shock. Therefore, the presence of shock in an injured patient demands the **immediate involvement of qualified surgeons.**

II. Hemorrhagic Shock in the Injured Patient

The trauma patient's response to blood loss is rendered more complex by changes in the body fluids (particularly in the extracellular fluid) that impact on the circulating blood volume and cellular function. The classic response to blood loss (described below) must be considered in the context of the fluid changes associated with soft tissue injury and the changes associated with severe, prolonged shock.

A. Pathophysiology

Early circulatory responses to blood loss are compensatory, ie, **progressive vasoconstriction** of cutaneous, visceral, and muscle circulation to preserve blood flow to the kidneys, heart, and brain. **Tachycardia** is the earliest measurable circulatory sign.

At the **cellular level**, inadequately perfused cells initially compensate by shifting to **anaerobic metabolism**, which further results in the formation of **lactic acid** and the development of **metabolic acidosis**. If shock is prolonged, cellular swelling occurs, leading to cellular damage and death, and tissue swelling. This process compounds the overall impact on blood loss and hypoperfusion. **The administration of isotonic electrolyte solutions helps combat this process. Therefore, management is directed toward reversing this cyclic phenomenon with adequate oxygenation, ventilation, and appropriate fluid resuscitation.**

B. Definition of Hemorrhage

Hemorrhage is defined as **an acute loss of circulating blood**. Normally, adult blood volume is approximately 7% of body weight. For example: a 70-kilogram male has approximately 5 liters of circulating blood volume. The blood volume of obese adults is estimated based on their ideal body weight, because calculation based on actual weight can result in significant overestimation. For children, the blood volume is calculated to be 8% to 9% of the body weight (80 to 90 ml/kg). (See Chapter 10—Pediatric Trauma.)

C. Direct Effect of Hemorrhage

Classes of hemorrhage, based on percentage of acute blood volume loss, are outlined individually in this chapter for the purposes of teaching and comprehending the physiologic and clinical manifestations of hemorrhagic shock. Class I is exemplified by the condition of the blood donor. **Class II** is uncomplicated shock, but fluid resuscitation is required. **Class III** is a complicated state in which at least crystalloid and perhaps blood replacement are required. **Class IV** can be considered as a preterminal event, and unless very aggressive measures are taken, the patient will be dead within minutes. (See Estimated Fluid and Blood Requirements chart at conclusion of this chapter.)

All medical personnel involved in the initial assessment and resuscitation of the patient in hemorrhagic shock must quickly recognize important factors that may accentuate or diminish the patient's physiologic response. Important factors that may profoundly alter the classic vascular dynamics include: 1) the patient's age; 2) severity of injury with special attention to type and anatomical location of injury; 3) time lapse between injury occurrence and initiation of treatment; and 4) prehospital fluid therapy and application of the pneumatic antishock garment (PASG).

It is dangerous to wait until the trauma patient fits a precise physiological classification of shock before initiating aggressive therapy. Aggressive fluid resuscitation must be initiated when early signs and symptoms of blood loss are apparent or suspected, not when the blood pressure is falling or absent.

1. Loss of up to 15%–Class I Hemorrhage

The clinical symptoms of this volume loss are minimal. In uncomplicated situations, minimal tachycardia occurs. No measurable changes occur in blood pressure, pulse pressure, respiratory rate, or capillary refill test. The capillary refill test is performed by depressing the fingernail or hypothenar eminence with the finger. A normal response is for the color to return within the period it takes for the examiner to say the phrase, "capillary return" (ie, two seconds). The capillary refill test cannot be interpreted in hypothermic patients. For otherwise healthy patients, this amount of blood loss does not require replacement. Transcapillary refill and other compensatory mechanisms restore blood volume within 24 hours. However, in the presence of other fluid changes, this amount of blood loss can produce clinical symptoms. Replacement of the primary fluid losses will correct the circulatory state.

2. 15% to 30% blood loss–Class II Hemorrhage

In a 70-kilogram male, this volume loss represents 800 to 1500 ml of blood. Clinical symptoms include tachycardia (heart rate above 100 in an adult), tachypnea, and a decrease in pulse pressure (the difference between the systolic and diastolic pressures). This decrease in pulse pressure is primarily related to a rise in diastolic component. (The main reason for the rise in diastolic pressure is an elevation in catecholamines which produces an increase in peripheral resistance). Because the systolic pressure changes minimally in early hemorrhagic shock, it is important to evaluate the pulse pressure rather than the systolic pressure. Other pertinent clinical findings with this degree of blood loss include subtle central nervous system changes (anxiety, which may be expressed as fright or hostility), and a positive capillary refill test. Notably, despite the significant blood loss and cardiovascular changes, urinary output is only mildly affected (the measured flow is usually 20 to 30 ml per hour).

Again, accompanying fluid losses can compound the clinical expression of this amount of blood loss. The majority of such patients may eventually require blood transfusion, but can be initially stabilized with other replacement fluids.

3. 30% to 40% blood volume loss–Class III Hemorrhage

This amount of blood loss (approximately 2000 ml in an adult) can be devastating. Patients almost always present with classical signs of inadequate perfusion, including marked tachycardia and tachypnea, significant changes in mental status, and a measurable fall in systolic pressure. Note that in an uncomplicated case, this is the smallest amount of blood loss that consistently causes a drop in systolic pressure. Although patients with this degree of blood loss will almost always require transfusion, remember that these symptoms can result from lesser degrees of blood loss combined with other fluid losses. Thus the decision to transfuse is based on the patient's response (as described later in this chapter).

4. More than 40% blood volume loss–Class IV Hemorrhage

This degree of exsanguination is immediately life-threatening. Symptoms include marked tachycardia, a significant depression in systolic blood pressure, and a very narrow pulse pressure (or an unobtainable diastolic pressure). Urinary output is negligible, and mental status is markedly depressed. The skin is cold and pale. Such patients frequently require rapid transfusion and immediate surgical intervention. These decisions are based on the patient's response to the initial management techniques described here. Loss of over 50% of the patient's blood volume results in loss of consciousness, pulse, and blood pressure.

D. Fluid Changes Secondary to Soft-Tissue Injury

Major soft-tissue injuries and fractures compound the circulatory status of the injured patient in two ways. First, blood is frequently lost into the site of injury, particularly in cases of major fractures. For instance, a fractured tibia or humerus may be associated with as much as a unit and a half (755 ml) blood loss. Twice that amount (up to 1500 ml) is commonly associated with femur fractures.

The second factor to be considered is the obligatory edema that occurs in injured soft tissues. This condition is related to the magnitude of soft-tissue injury and consists of extracellular fluid. Because the plasma acts as part of the extracellular fluid, these changes have a significant impact on circulating blood volume. For instance, the two liters of edema that may be associated with a massive femur fracture would be represented by 1500 ml of interstitial fluid and 500 ml of plasma volume. In general, roughly 25% of such fluid translocation will be evidenced by a decrease in the plasma volume. The impact of these changes on circulating blood volume and the reason they compound fluid loss then becomes obvious.

III. Initial Patient Assessment

A. Recognition of Shock

Full-blown circulatory shock, evidenced by inadequate perfusion of the skin, kidneys, and central nervous system, is easy to recognize. However, after the airway and breathing are evaluated, careful evaluation of the patient's circulatory status is important to identify earlier stages of shock. **Remember, compensatory mechanisms may have precluded a measurable fall in systolic pressure until the patient has lost up to 30% of his blood volume.** Specific attention should be directed to pulse rate, respiratory rate, skin circulation, and **pulse pressure. A narrowed pulse pressure** suggests significant blood loss and involvement of compensatory mechanisms. The earliest signs of shock are tachycardia and cutaneous vasoconstriction. **Accordingly, any injured patient who is cool and tachycardic is in shock until proven otherwise.** The normal heart rate varies with age. Tachycardia is present when the heart rate is greater than 160 in an infant; 140 in a preschool age child; 120 from school age to puberty; 100 in an adult. The elderly patient may not exhibit tachycardia because of a limited cardiac response to catecholamine stimulation or certain medications such as propanolol.

Use of the hematocrit (or hemoglobin concentration) is unreliable and inappropriate for estimating acute blood loss or diagnosing shock. Massive blood loss may produce a minimal acute decrease in hematocrit. Thus a very low hematocrit suggests significant blood loss or pre-existing anemia, while a near normal hematocrit does **not** rule out significant blood loss.

B. Clinical Differentiation of Etiology

Hemorrhage is the most common cause of shock after injury, and virtually all multiply injured patients have an element of hypovolemia. Therefore, once the shock state is identified, treatment is usually begun as if the patient were hypovolemic. As this treatment is instituted, it is important to identify the small number of patients whose shock has been caused by some other etiology, and the larger group of patients for whom a secondary factor complicates their hypovolemic shock. **The major differentiating factor in identifying the cause of shock in a trauma patient is whether the condition is hypovolemic or cardiogenic, especially for a patient with injuries above the diaphragm. A high index of suspicion and careful observation of the patient's response to treatment should enable the physician to recognize and manage all forms of shock. The initial determination of the etiology depends on an appropriate history, a careful physical examination, and selected additional tests.**

1. Cardiogenic shock

Myocardial dysfunction may occur from tension pneumothorax, myocardial contusion, cardiac tamponade, air embolus, or rarely a myocardial infarction associated with the patient's injury. Cardiac contusion is not uncommon in rapid deceleration blunt trauma to the thorax. All patients with blunt thoracic trauma need constant ECG monitoring to detect injury patterns and dysrhythmias. Blood CPK and isoenzymes should be drawn on admission, but rarely have any value in diagnosing or managing the patient in the emergency room. Ultrasound and specific isotope studies of the myocardium are not practical tests for the emergency room. Myocardial contusion may be an indication for early central venous pressure monitoring of fluid resuscitation in the emergency department.

Cardiac tamponade is most common in penetrating thoracic trauma. It can occur rarely in blunt trauma to the thorax or in a patient who had myocardial infarction with tamponade as a cause or result of the accident. Tachycardia; muffled heart sounds; and dilated, engorged neck veins with hypotension resistant to fluid therapy suggest cardiac tamponade. The only condition that mimics cardiac tamponade is tension pneumothorax. Appropriate placement of a needle temporarily relieves these two life-threatening conditions.

2. Neurogenic shock

Isolated head injuries do not cause shock. The presence of shock in a patient with a head injury indicates a search for another cause of shock. Spinal cord injury may produce hypotension due to loss of sympathetic tone. **Remember, loss of sympathetic tone compounds the physiologic effects of hypovolemia, and hypovolemia compounds the physiologic effects of sympathetic denervation.** The classic picture of neurogenic shock is hypotension without tachycardia or cutaneous vasoconstriction. Patients with known or suspected neurogenic shock should be treated initially for hypovolemia. Vasoactive drugs should **not** be administered until volume is restored. Venous pressure monitoring is extremely helpful in managing this sometimes complex problem.

3. Septic shock

Shock due to infection immediately after injury is uncommon. However, if the patient's arrival at the emergency facility is delayed for several hours, this problem may occur. Septic shock is particularly likely to occur in patients with penetrating abdominal injuries and contamination of the peritoneal cavity with intestinal contents. The volume status of the patient in septic shock is clinically significant. Septic patients who are hypovolemic are difficult to distinguish clinically from those in hypovolemic shock (tachycardia, cutaneous vasoconstriction, impaired urinary output, decreased systolic pressure, narrow pulse pressure). Patients with sepsis and normal or nearly normal circulating volume may have a modest tachycardia, warm pink skin, a systolic pressure near normal, and a **wide pulse pressure.**

IV. Initial Management of Hemorrhagic Shock

As in many emergency situations, diagnosis and treatment must be performed in rapid succession. For most trauma patients, treatment is instituted as if the patient had hypovolemic shock, unless evidence to the contrary is clear.

A. Physical Examination

The physical examination is directed at the immediate diagnosis of life-threatening injuries and includes assessment of the ABCs. Baseline recordings are important to the subsequent monitoring of the patient. Vital signs, urinary output, and level of consciousness are important. A more detailed examination of the patient follows as the situation permits.

1. Airway–Breathing

The adequacy of ventilation is assessed. Establishing a patent airway with adequate ventilatory exchange is the first priority. After establishing an adequate airway, oxygen is administered. Supplementary oxygen via a bag-valve-mask reservoir system is delivered to maintain arterial oxygen tension between 80 and 100 mmHg.

2. Bleeding–Hemorrhage control

Bleeding from external wounds usually can be controlled by direct pressure to the bleeding site, eg, scalp, neck, and upper and lower extremity. Pneumatic antishock trousers may be used to control bleeding from pelvic and open lower extremity fractures. However, this device should **not** interfere with rapid re-establishment of intravascular volume by the intravenous route.

3. Gastric dilatation–Decompression

Gastric dilatation often occurs in the trauma victim in spite of a nasogastric tube. **This condition makes shock difficult to treat, and the unconscious patient is always in danger of aspiration, a potentially fatal complication.** The physician's responsibility does not end with the passage of the tube. The tube must be properly positioned, attached to appropriate suction, and be functioning.

B. Vascular Access Lines

Access to the vascular system must be obtained promptly. This is best done by establishing two large-bore (#16-gauge or larger) catheters before any consideration is given to a central line. The most desirable sites for peripheral intravenous lines (in order of priority) are: 1) percutaneous peripheral access via forearm or antecubital veins, and 2) cutdown on the saphenous or arm veins. If circumstances prevent the use of peripheral veins, central venous access is indicated, using the Seldinger technique.

As the intravenous lines are started, blood samples are drawn for appropriate laboratory analyses, type and crossmatch, and toxicology. It also may be useful to obtain arterial blood gases at this time.

C. Initial Fluid Therapy

Isotonic electrolyte solutions are used for initial resuscitation. This type of fluid provides transient intravascular expansion and further stabilizes the vascular volume by replacing accompanying fluid losses. Ringer's lactate solution is the initial fluid of choice. Normal saline is the second choice. Although normal saline is a satisfactory replacement fluid in the volumes administered to injured patients, it has the potential to cause hyperchloremic acidosis. This potential is enhanced if renal function is impaired.

An initial fluid bolus is given as rapidly as possible. The usual dose is one to two liters for an adult and 20 ml/kilogram for a pediatric patient. The patient's response is observed during this initial fluid administration, and further therapeutic and diagnostic decisions are based on this response.

The amount of fluid and blood required for resuscitation is difficult to predict on initial evaluation of the patient. However, general guidelines are available for establishing the amount and type of fluid and blood the patient will probably require. If, during resuscitation, the amounts administered deviate widely from these estimates, a careful reassessment of the situation and a search for unrecognized injuries or other causes of shock are necessary. (See Table 1–Estimated Fluid and Blood Requirements, at conclusion of this chapter.)

V. Evaluation of Response/Continued Therapy

A. General

The same signs and symptoms of inadequate perfusion that were used to diagnose shock are useful determiners of patient response. The return of normal blood pressure, pulse pressure, and pulse rate are positive signs, and indicate that circulation is stabilizing. However, these observations give no information regarding organ perfusion. Improvements in the central nervous system status and skin circulation are important evidence of enhanced perfusion, but are difficult to quantitate. The urinary output can be quantitated and the renal response to restoration of perfusion is reasonably sensitive (if not modified by diuretics). For this reason urinary output is one of the prime monitors of resuscitation and patient response. Changes in central venous pressure can provide useful information, and the risk of a central venous pressure line is justified for complex cases. Measurements of left heart function (obtained with a Swan-Ganz catheter) are rarely indicated for the emergency room management of the injured patient.

B. Urinary Output

Within certain limits, urinary output can be used as a monitor of renal blood flow. **Adequate volume replacement should produce a urinary output of approximately 50 ml/hour in the adult. One ml/ kg/hour** is an adequate urinary output for the **pediatric patient.** For children under one year of age, two ml/kg/hour should be maintained. Inability to obtain urinary output at these levels (or decreasing urinary output with an increasing specific gravity) suggests inadequate resuscitation. This situation should stimulate further volume replacement and diagnostic endeavors.

C. Acid/Base Balance

Patients in early hypovolemic shock have respiratory alkalosis due to tachypnea. Respiratory alkalosis gives way to a mild metabolic acidosis in the early phases of shock, and does not require treatment. Severe metabolic acidosis may develop from long-standing or severe shock. Metabolic acidosis is due to anaerobic metabolism resulting from inadequate tissue perfusion, and persistence is usually due to inadequate fluid resuscitation. Persistent acidosis in the normothermic shock patient should be treated with increased fluids and not intravenous sodium bicarbonate, unless the pH is less than 7.2.

VI. Therapeutic Decisions

Having established a preliminary plan based on the initial evaluation of the patient, the physician can now modify management, depending on the patient's response to initial resuscitative fluids. This approach identifies those patients whose blood loss was greater than estimated and those with ongoing bleeding. In addition, it limits the probability of overtransfusion or unneeded transfusion of blood in those whose initial status was disproportionate to the amount of blood loss. The potential response patterns can be discussed in three groups.

A. Rapid Response to Initial Fluid Administration

A small group of patients will respond rapidly to the initial fluid bolus, and will remain stable when the initial fluid has been completed and the fluids are slowed. Such patients will usually have lost less than 20% of their blood volume. No further fluid bolus or immediate blood administration is indicated for this small group of patients. Type and crossmatched blood should be kept available. **Surgical consultation and evaluation are necessary during initial assessment and treatment.**

B. Transient Response to Initial Fluid Administration

The largest group of patients will respond to the initial fluid bolus. However, as the initial fluids are slowed, the circulatory perfusion indices will begin to show deterioration in these patients (most of whom will have lost 20% to 40% of their blood volume or who are still bleeding). Continued fluid administration and initiation of blood administration are indicated. The response to blood administration should identify patients who are still bleeding and require **rapid surgical intervention.**

C. Minimal or No Response to Initial Fluid Administration

This response is seen in a small but significant percentage of injured patients. For most of these patients, failure to respond to adequate crystalloid and blood administration in the emergency department dictates the need for immediate surgical intervention to control exsanguinating hemorrhage. On very rare occasions, failure to respond may be due to pump failure as a result of myocardial contusion or cardiac tamponade. Central venous pressure monitoring helps differentiate between these two groups of patients.

VII. Blood Replacement

The decision to begin transfusion is based on the patient's response, as described in the previous section.

A. Crossmatched, Type-Specific, and Type O Blood

1. Fully crossmatched blood is preferable. However, the complete crossmatching procedure requires approximately an hour in most blood banks. For patients who stabilize rapidly, crossmatched blood should be obtained and be available for transfusion when indicated.

2. Type-specific or "saline crossmatched" blood can be provided by most blood banks within ten minutes. Such blood is compatible with ABO and Rh blood types. Incompatibilities of minor antibodies may exist. Such blood is of first choice for patients with life-threatening shock situations, such as transient responders described in the previous section.

3. If type-specific blood is **unavailable,** type O packed cells are indicated for patients with **exsanguinating hemorrhage.** To avoid sensitization and future complications, Rh-negative cells are preferable, particularly for women of child-bearing age.

B. Blood Filters

Macropore (160 microns) intravenous filtering devices are used when whole blood transfusions are given. These filters remove microscopic clots and debris. The use of micropore blood filters has not been demonstrated to be of significant value.

C. Warming Fluids–Plasma and Crystalloid

Iatrogenic hypothermia in the resuscitation phase of trauma victims can and **must be prevented.** The use of blood warmers is cumbersome yet most desirable in the emergency department. The most efficient and easy way to prevent hypothermia in any patient receiving massive volumes of crystalloid is to heat the fluid to 39 ° C before using it. Blood, plasma, and glucose-containing solutions cannot be warmed in the microwave oven.

D. Coagulopathy

Coagulopathy is a rare problem in the first hour of treatment of the multiply injured patient. Prothrombin time, partial thromboplastin time, and platelet count are valuable baseline studies to obtain in the first hour, especially if the patient has a history of coagulation disorders or takes medications that alter coagulation. Routine use of fresh frozen plasma and platelets in patients with dilutional coagulopathy after massive fluid and blood replacement is costly, dangerous, and unwarranted.

E. Calcium Administration

The majority of the patients receiving blood transfusions do not need calcium supplements in the first hour of treatment.

VIII. Pneumatic Antishock Garment (PASG)

The application of the PASG can raise systolic pressure by increasing peripheral vascular resistance and myocardial afterload. Use of the PASG is controversial. If the need for application has been recognized during the delivery of prehospital care, most patients will arrive in the emergency department with the PASG applied.

A. Indications

Current indications for **inhospital** use of the PASG are:

1. Splinting and control of pelvic fractures with **continuing hemorrhage and hypotension.**

2. Intra-abdominal trauma with severe hypovolemia in patients who are en route to the operating room or another facility. A number of investigative studies suggest that the garment may reduce intra-abdominal hemorrhage.

B. Contraindications

1. Uncontrolled hemorrhage outside the confines of the garment is a relative contraindication.

2. Pulmonary edema, known rupture of the diaphragm, and left ventricular dysfunction are absolute contraindications.

C. Dangers

The use of the PASG **must not delay volume replacement or rapid transport for penetrating trauma.** Precise time that the leg compartments have been inflated must be documented on the patient's records. **Any patient with extremity trauma and associated history of shock should not have the leg segments inflated for prolonged periods of time.**

If inflation of the abdominal component of the PASG causes an increase in the patient's respiratory rate or respiratory distress, it must be deflated immediately, regardless of the patient's blood pressure. Diaphragmatic rupture is assumed until proven otherwise.

D. Deflation and Removal of PASG

Several specific points bear emphasis in deflation procedures. The trousers can be removed after the shock state is adequately managed, and vital signs are within acceptable limits. Individual segments may be carefully deflated for examination of extremities, angiography, etc. In general, if the patient requires transfer to another facility, the garment is left inflated. For patients transferred by air, effective inflation pressures may increase due to changes in atmospheric pressure. A similar change may occur when the PASG is applied in a cold environment, and the patient is then brought into a warm emergency department.

The deflation process is gradual. Deflation of the garment begins with the waist or abdominal segment. A small amount of air is allowed to escape from the valve, while the patient's blood pressure is carefully monitored. Deflation is continued until the patient exhibits a blood pressure drop of 5 mmHg. At this point, deflation is stopped, and intravenous fluid replacement is increased until the blood pressure returns to normal limits. Deflation is resumed. When the abdominal segment has been deflated, the legs are sequentially deflated, carefully monitoring the patient's blood pressure.

IX. Pitfalls in the Diagnosis and Treatment of Shock

A. Age

The older patient has difficulty tolerating hypotension from hemorrhage due to trauma. Aggressive therapy with fluids and early surgery are often warranted to save the patient and prevent serious complications, such as myocardial infarction or a cerebrovascular accident.

B. Athletes

Rigorous training routines change the cardiovascular dynamics of this group of patients. Blood volume can increase 15% to 20%, cardiac outputs can increase six-fold, stroke volume can increase 50%, and resting pulse is generally at 50. This group's ability to compensate for blood loss is truly remarkable. Any athlete with suspected hemorrhage due to trauma must be watched carefully.

C. Medications

Beta-adrenergic receptor blockers and calcium antagonists can significantly alter the patient's hemodynamic response to hemorrhage.

D. Hypothermia

Body temperature is one of the most important vital signs recorded in the initial assessment phase. Theoretically, esophageal recording is the most accurate measurement of the core temperature. Although not ideal, a rectal temperature will alert the treating physician to the problem. A trauma victim under the influence of alcohol and exposed to cold temperature extremes may become hypothermic. Patients suffering from hypothermia and hemorrhagic shock are resistant to appropriate blood and fluid resuscitative measures and surgical treatment. The only true indication for vasopressors in hypovolemic shock is the hypothermic trauma patient who sustains a cardiac arrest. Rapid rewarming with an appropriate warming blanket, warm fluids, and blood generally corrects the patient's hypotension and hypothermia.

E. Pacemaker

About 150,000 such devices are placed in patients with myocardial conduction defects every year in North America. These patients are unable to respond to blood loss in the expected fashion. For this group, central venous pressure monitoring is invaluable to guide fluid therapy.

X. Avoiding Complications

Inadequate volume replacement with subsequent organ failure is the most common complication of hemorrhagic shock. Immediate, appropriate, and aggressive therapy that restores organ perfusion will minimize these untoward events. Three specific concerns are outlined in the succeeding paragraphs.

A. Continued Hemorrhage

Obscure hemorrhage is the most common cause of poor patient response to fluid therapy. Under this circumstance, consider **immediate surgical intervention.**

B. Fluid Overload and CVP Monitoring

After the patient's initial assessment and management has been completed, the risk of fluid overload is minimized by monitoring the patient carefully. **Remember, the goal of therapy is restoration of organ perfusion,** signified by appropriate urinary output, central nervous system function, skin color, and return of pulse and blood pressure toward normal.

Central venous pressure monitoring is a relatively simple procedure and is used as a standard guide for assessing the right heart's ability to accept a fluid load. Properly interpreted, the response of the central venous pressure to fluid administration helps evaluate volume replacement. Several points to remember are:

1. The precise measure of cardiac function is the relationship between ventricular-end diastolic volume and stroke volume. It is apparent that comparison of right atrial pressure (CVP) to cardiac output (as reflected by evidence of perfusion or blood pressure, or even by direct measurement), is an indirect and, at best, an insensitive estimate of this relationtship. The CVP is valid for gross evaluation of appropriate clinical situations. Remembering these facts is important to avoid overdependence on CVP monitoring.

2. The initial central venous pressure level and the actual blood volume are not necessarily related. The initial central venous pressure is sometimes high even with a significant volume deficit, especially in patients with generalized vasoconstriction and rapid fluid replacement. The initial venous pressure may also be high secondary to the application of the PASG or the inappropriate use of exogenous vasopressors.

3. A minimal rise in the initial, low central venous pressure with fluid therapy suggests the need for further volume expansion.

4. A declining central venous pressure suggests ongoing fluid loss and the need for additional fluid or blood replacement.

5. An abrupt or persistent elevation in the central venous pressure suggests volume replacement has been adequate, is too rapid, or that cardiac function has been compromised.

6. **Remember,** the central venous pressure line is not a primary intravenous fluid resuscitation route. It should be inserted on an elective rather than emergent basis.

7. Pronounced elevations of the central venous pressure may be caused by catheter malposition, hypervolemia as a result of overtransfusion, cardiac dysfunction, or cardiac tamponade. Increased intrathoracic pressure from a pneumothorax may also cause an elevation in the central venous pressure.

Access for a central venous pressure line is through the antecubital, internal jugular, or subclavian veins. Appropriate antiseptic techniques are used when central lines are placed. Ideal placement of an intravenous catheter is in the superior vena cava, just proximal to the right atrium. Techniques will be discussed in detail in Skill Station IV—Percutaneous Venous Access.

Central venous lines are not without complications. Infections, vascular injury, embolization, thrombosis, and pneumothorax are encountered. Central venous pressure monitoring reflects right heart function. It may not be representative of the left heart function in patients with primary myocardial dysfunction or abnormal pulmonary circulation.

C. Recognition of Other Problems

When the patient **fails to respond** to therapy, consider ventilatory problems, unrecognized fluid loss, acute gastric distention, cardiac tamponade, myocardial infarction, diabetic acidosis, hypoadrenalism, and neurogenic shock. **Constant re-evaluation,** especially when patients deviate from expected patterns, is the key to recognizing such problems as early as possible.

XI. Summary

Shock therapy, based on sound physiological principles, is usually successful. Hypovolemia is the cause of shock in most trauma patients. Management of these patients requires immediate hemorrhage control and fluid replacement. Other possible causes of the shock state must be considered. The patient's response to initial fluid therapy determines further therapeutic and diagnostic procedures. The goal of therapy is restoration of organ perfusion. In hypovolemic shock, vasopressors are rarely, if ever, needed. Central venous pressure measurement is a valuable tool for confirming the volume status and monitoring the rate of fluid administration.

Table 1
Estimated Fluid and Blood Requirements[1]
(Based on Patient's Initial Presentation)

	Class I	Class II	Class III	Class IV
Blood Loss (ml)	up to 750	750-1500	1500-2000	2000 or more
Blood Loss (%BV)	up to 15%	15–30%	30–40%	40% or more
Pulse Rate	< 100	> 100	> 120	140 or higher
Blood Pressure	Normal	Normal	Decreased	Decreased
Pulse Pressure (mmHG)	Normal or increased	Decreased	Decreased	Decreased
Capillary Refill Test	Normal	Positive	Positive	Positive
Respiratory Rate	14–20	20–30	30–40	> 35
Urine Output (ml/hr)	30 or more	20–30	5–15	Negligible
CNS–Mental Status	Slightly anxious	Mildly anxious	Anxious and confused	Confused - lethargic
Fluid Replacement (3:1 Rule)	Crystalloid	Crystalloid	Crystalloid + blood	Crystalloid + blood

[1] For a 70-kg male

The guidelines in Table 1 are based on the **"three-for-one" rule.** This rule derives from the empiric observation that most patients in hemorrhagic shock will require as much as 300 ml of electrolyte solution for each 100 ml of blood loss. Applied blindly, these guidelines can result in excessive or inadequate fluid administration. For example, a patient with a crush injury to the extremity will have hypotension out of proportion to his blood loss and will require fluids in excess of the 3:1 guidelines. In contrast, a patient whose ongoing blood loss is being replaced will require less than 3:1. The use of bolus therapy with careful monitoring of the patient's response can moderate these extremes. (See Chapter 3—Shock, "Therapeutic Decisions".)

Bibliography

1. Carrico CJ, Canizaro PC, Shires GT: Fluid Resuscitation Following Injury: rationale for the use of balanced salt solutions. **Critical Care Medicine** 1976; 4(2):46-54.

2. Cogbill TH, Blintz M, Johnson JA, et al: Acute Gastric Dilatation after Trauma. **The Journal of Trauma** 1987; 27(10):1113- 1117.

3. Counts RB, Haisch C, Simon TL, et al: Hemostasis in Massively Transfused Trauma Patients.**Annals of Surgery** 1979;190(1): 91-99.

4. Demling RH, Duy N, Manohar M, Proctor R: Comparison Between Lung Fluid Filtration Rate and Measured Starling Forces after Hemorrhagic and Endotoxic Shock. **The Journal of Trauma** 1980;20(10):856-860.

5. Harrigan C, Lucas CE, Ledgerwood AM, et al: Several Changes in Primary Hemostasis after Massive Transfusion. **Surgery** 1985;98:836-840.

6. Martin DJ, Lucas CE, Ledgerwood AM, et al: Fresh Frozen Plasma Supplement to Massive Red Blood Cell Transfusion. **Annals of Surgery** 1985;202:505.

7. Poole GV, Meredith JW, Pennell T, et al: Comparison of Colloids and Crystalloids in Resuscitation from Hemorrhagic Shock. **Surgery, Gynecology and Obstetrics** 1982;154:577-586.

8. Schwab CW, Gore D: MAST: Medical Antishock Trousers in Nyhus L (ed): **Surgery Annual** Volume 15. Norwalk, Connecticut, Appleton- Centruy-Crofts, 1983; pp 41-59.

9. Schwartz SI: Hemostasis, Surgical Bleeding and Transfusion, in Schwartz S (ed): **Principles of Surgery, 4th Edition**. New York, McGraw-Hill, 1984; pp 81-114.

10. Virgilio RW, Rice CL, Smith DE, et al: Crystalloid vs Colloid Resuscitation: Is one Better? A randomized clinical study. **Surgery 85** February 1979, pp 129- 139.

11. Werwath DL, Schwab CW, Scholter JR, Robinett W: Microwave Ovens: A Safe New Method of Warming Crystalloids. **American Journal of Surgery** December 1984, pp 656-659.

Chapter 3:
Shock

Skill Station IV:
Percutaneous Venous Access

Equipment

1. Live patient model
2. Central venous pressure set-up
3. Subclavian intravenous set-up
4. Needles/intravenous catheters
   a. Assorted intravenous over-the-needle catheters (#14-, #16-, and #18-gauge, 15-20 cm in length)
   b. #18-gauge needle (1.5 inches in length)
   c. #19-gauge needle (1.5 inches in length)
   d. J-wire
5. Antiseptic swabs
6. 6-ml syringes
7. Lidocaine 1% (demonstration purposes only)
8. 250 ml, 5% D/W with macrodrip
9. Large caliber intravenous and extension tubings
10. Portable intravenous stand (optional)
11. 3x3s

Objectives

1. Performance at this station will allow the participant to practice and demonstrate the technique of subclavian and internal jugular intravenous line insertions.

2. Upon completion of this station, the participant will be able to describe the surface markings for insertion of an intravenous catheter into a:

   a. Subclavian vein
   b. Internal jugular vein
   c. Femoral vein

3. Upon completion of this station, the participant will be able to identify the intravenous fluid used for the following types of shock and associated trauma:

   a. Hypovolemic shock
   b. Cardiogenic shock
   c. Septic shock
   d. Neurogenic shock

1. Subclavian venipuncture: infraclavicular approach

Procedures

2. Internal jugular venipuncture

3. Femoral venipuncture

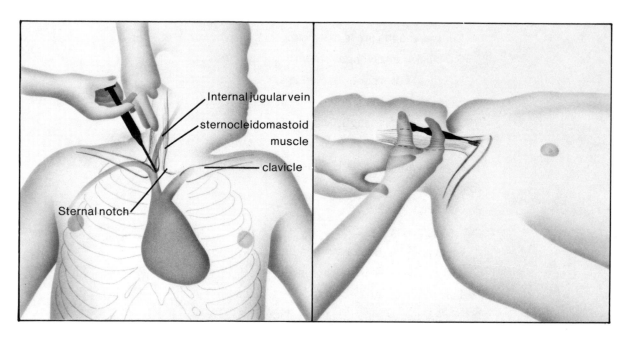

Internal Jugular Venipuncture: Middle or Central Route

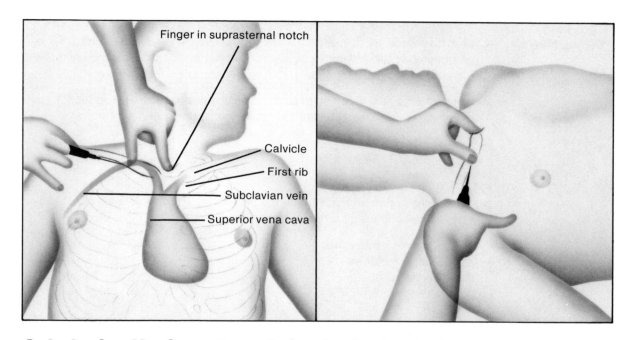

Subclavian Venipuncture: Infraclavicular Approach

Skills Procedures

Percutaneous Venous Access

I. Subclavian Venipuncture–Infraclavicular Approach

A. Place the patient in a supine position, at least 15 degrees head-down to distend the neck veins and prevent an air embolism. Turn the patient's head away from the venipuncture site.

B. Cleanse the skin well around the venipuncture site and drape the area. Sterile gloves should be worn when performing this procedure.

C. If the patient is awake, use a local anesthetic at the venipuncture site.

D. Introduce a large-caliber needle, attached to a 6-ml syringe with 0.5 ml to 1 ml saline, 1 cm below the junction of the middle and medial thirds of the clavicle.

E. After the skin has been punctured, with the bevel of the needle upward, expel the skin plug that may occlude the needle.

F. The needle and syringe are held parallel to the frontal plane.

G. Direct the needle medially, slightly cephaled, and posteriorly behind the clavicle toward the posterior, superior angle of the sternal end of the clavicle (toward finger placed in the suprasternal notch).

H. Slowly advance the needle while gently withdrawing the plunger of the syringe.

I. When a free flow of blood appears in the syringe, rotate the bevel of the needle caudally, remove the syringe, and occlude the needle with a finger to prevent an air embolism.

J. Quickly insert the catheter to a predetermined depth (tip of catheter should be above the right atrium for fluid administration).

K. Remove the needle and connect the catheter to the intravenous tubing.

L. Affix the catheter (eg, with suture), apply antibiotic ointment, and dress the area.

M. Tape the intravenous tubing in place.

N. Attach the central venous pressure set-up to the intravenous tubing and adjust the manometer (level at zero) with the level of the patient's right atrium.

O. Obtain a chest film to ascertain position of intravenous line and possible pneumothorax.

II. Internal Jugular Venipuncture–Middle or Central Route

A. Place the patient in a supine position, at least 15 degrees head-down to distend the neck veins and to prevent an air embolism. Turn the patient's head away from the venipuncture site.

B. Cleanse the skin well around the venipuncture site and drape the area. Sterile gloves should be worn when performing this procedure.

C. If the patient is awake, use a local anesthetic at the venipuncture site.

D. Introduce a large-caliber needle, attached to a 6-ml syringe with 0.5 ml to 1 ml of saline, into the center of the triangle formed by the two lower heads of the sternomastoid and the clavicle.

E. After the skin has been punctured, with the bevel of the needle upward, expel the skin plug that may occlude the needle.

F. Direct the needle caudally, parallel to the sagittal plane, at a 30-degree posterior angle with the frontal plane.

G. Slowly advance the needle while gently withdrawing the plunger of the syringe.

H. When a free flow of blood appears in the syringe, remove the syringe and occlude the needle with a finger to prevent an air embolism. If the vein is not entered, withdraw the needle and redirect it 5 degrees to 10 degrees laterally.

I. Quickly insert the catheter to a predetermined depth (tip of catheter should be above the right atrium for fluid administration).

J. Remove the needle and connect the catheter to the intravenous tubing.

K. Affix the catheter in place (eg, with suture), apply antibiotic ointment, and dress the area.

L. Tape the intravenous tubing in place.

M. Attach the central venous pressure setup to the intravenous tubing and adjust the manometer (level at zero) with the level of the patient's right atrium.

N. Obtain a chest film to ascertain position of the intravenous line and possible pneumothorax.

Complications of Central Intravenous Venipuncture

1. Hematoma formation
2. Cellulitis
3. Thrombosis
4. Phlebitis
5. Nerve transection
6. Arterial puncture
7. Pneumothorax
8. Hemopneumothorax (eg, with subclavian venipuncture)
9. Nerve puncture
10. Chylothorax (eg, with internal jugular venipuncture)

11. Arteriovenous fistula
12. Peripheral neuropathy
13. Lost catheters
14. Inaccurate monitoring techniques
15. Improperly placed catheters

III. Femoral Venipuncture

A. Place the patient in a supine position.

B. Cleanse the skin well around the venipuncture site and drape the area. Sterile gloves should be worn when performing this procedure.

C. Locate the femoral vein by palpating the femoral artery. The vein lies directly medial to the femoral artery (nerve, artery, vein, empty space). A finger should remain on the artery to facilitate anatomical location, and to avoid insertion of the catheter into the artery.

D. If the patient is awake, use a local anesthetic at the venipuncture site.

E. Introduce a #19-gauge needle, attached to a 6-ml syringe with 0.5 to 1 ml of saline. The needle, directed towards the patient's head, should enter the skin directly over the femoral vein.

F. The needle and syringe are held parallel to the frontal plane.

G. Directing the needle cephaled and posteriorly, slowly advance the needle while gently withdrawing the plunger of the syringe.

H. When a free flow of blood appears in the syringe, remove the syringe and occlude the needle with a finger to prevent air embolism.

I. Insert the guidewire and remove the needle. Then insert the catheter over the guidewire.

J. Remove the guidewire and needle, and connect the catheter to the intravenous tubing.

K. Affix the catheter in place (ie, with suture), apply antibiotic ointment, and dress the area.

L. Tape the intravenous tubing in place.

M. Attach the central venous pressure setup to the intravenous tubing and adjust the manometer (level at zero) with the level of the patient's right atrium.

N. Obtain chest and abdominal roentgenograms to ascertain position and placement of the intravenous catheter.

Complications of Femoral Venipuncture

1. Hematoma formation
2. Cellulitis
3. Thrombosis
4. Phlebitis

5. Nerve transection and/or puncture
6. Arterial puncture
7. Arteriovenous fistula
8. Peripheral neuropathy
9. Lost catheters
10. Inaccurate monitoring techniques
11. Improperly placed catheter

Skill Station V:
Venous Cutdown

This surgical procedure, if performed on a live, anesthetized animal, must be conducted in a USDA Registered Animal Laboratory. (See *ATLS Instructor Manual*, Section II, Chapter 10—Animal Laboratory Guidelines and Protocols.)

Equipment

1. Live, anesthetized animals

2. Licensed veterinarian (see guidelines referenced above)

3. Animal troughs, ropes (sandbags optional)

4. Animal intubation equipment

    a. Endotracheal tubes

    b. Laryngoscope blade and handle

    c. Respirator with 15-mm adapter

5. Electric shears with #40 blade

6. Local anesthetic set, including antiseptic

7. Tables or instrument stands

8. #14- to #20-gauge cutdown catheters

9. Suture

    a. 3-0 ties

    b. 4-0 suture with swaged needle

10. Surgical instruments

    a. Scalpel handles with #10 and #11 blades

    b. Small hemostats

    c. Needle holders

    d. Single-toothed spring retractors

11. 4x4s

12. Surgical drapes

13. 500-ml Ringer's lactate with macrodrip tubing

14. Vein introducer (optional)

15. Surgical garb (gloves, shoe covers, and scrub suits or cover gowns)

1. Performance at this station will allow the participant to practice and demonstrate on a live anesthetized animal the technique of peripheral venous cutdown. **Objectives**

2. Upon completion of this station, the participant will be able to identify the surface markings and structures to be noted in performing a peripheral venous cutdown.

3. Upon completion of this station, the participant will be able to discuss the indications and contraindications for a peripheral venous cutdown.

Anatomical Considerations for Venous Cutdown

1. The primary site for a peripheral venous cutdown is the greater saphenous vein at the ankle, which is located at a point approximately 2 cm anterior and superior to the medial malleolus.

2. A secondary site is the antecubital medial basilic vein, located 2.5 cm lateral to the medial epicondyle of the humerus at the flexion crease of the elbow.

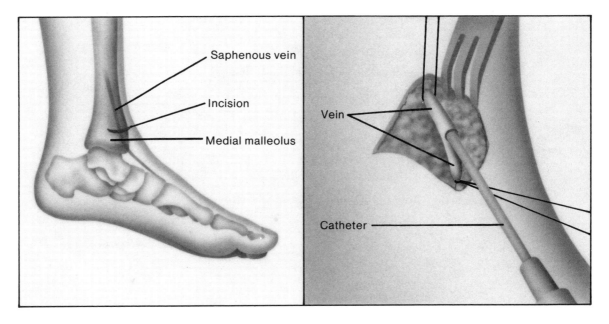

Saphenous Venous Cutdown

Skills Procedure

Venous Cutdown

I. Venous Cutdown

A. Prepare the skin of the ankle with an antiseptic solution and drape the area.

B. Infiltrate the skin over the vein with 0.5% lidocaine.

C. A full-thickness transverse skin incision is made through the area of anesthesia to a length of 2.5 cm.

D. By blunt dissection, using a curved hemostat, the vein is identified and dissected free from any accompanying structures.

E. Elevate and dissect the vein for a distance of approximately 2 cm, to free it from its bed.

F. Ligate the distal, mobilized vein, leaving the suture in place for traction.

G. Pass a tie about the vein, cephaled.

H. Make a small transverse venotomy and gently dilate the venotomy with the tip of a closed hemostat.

I. Introduce a plastic cannula through the venotomy and secure it in place by tying the upper ligature about the vein and cannula. The cannula should be inserted an adequate distance to prevent disloding.

J. Attach the intravenous tubing to the cannula and close the incision with interrupted sutures.

K. Apply a sterile dressing with a topical antibiotic ointment.

Complications of Peripheral Venous Cutdown

1. Cellulitis
2. Hematoma
3. Phlebitis
4. Perforation of the posterior wall of the vein
5. Venous thrombosis
6. Nerve transection
7. Arterial transection

**Chapter 3:
Shock**

**Skill
Station
V**

American College of Surgeons

Skill Station VI: Application of Pneumatic Antishock Garment

Equipment

1. Pneumatic antishock garment (type commonly used in locale)
2. Blood pressure cuff
3. Stethoscope
4. Resusci-Anne II
5. Long spine board

Caution: When these trousers are demonstrated on live models (non-patients), they should never be inflated to avoid the possibility of untoward blood pressure elevations.

Objectives

1. Performance at this station enables the participant to practice and demonstrate the proper technique for applying the pneumatic antishock garment.

2. Upon completion of this station, the participant will be able to demonstrate the method for proper inflation and deflation of the pneumatic antishock garment.

3. Upon completion of this station, the participant will be able to discuss the rationale for the use of the pneumatic antishock garment including the indications for inhospital use and contraindications.

**Chapter 3:
Shock**

**Skill
Station
VI**

American College of Surgeons

Pneumatic Antishock Garment

I. Application of the Pneumatic Antishock Garment

A. Application

1. Record the patient's vital signs.

2. Unfold the trousers and lay flat on the long spine board.

3. Carefully slide the trousers with the spine board under the patient, maintaining immobility of the spine.

4. Fold the trousers about the left leg first and fasten.

5. Fold the trousers about the right leg and fasten.

6. Fold the trousers about the abdomen and fasten.

7. Attach the air tubes to the connections on the pants. Be sure all stopcocks are open.

B. Inflation

1. Recheck the vital signs.

2. Inflate the legs first and the abdomen last.

3. Determine the amount of inflation necessary by the patient's perfusion status. **Inflation should stop when the patient's blood pressure or perfusion status has reached an acceptable level.**

4. When the optimal blood pressure is obtained, turn the stopcocks to the hold position.

5. **Do not inflate the trousers on the basis of pressure readings in the trousers themselves, but on the basis of the patient's blood pressure.**

6. Monitor the **patient's** blood pressure and add pressure to the trousers, asneeded, to maintain an optimal pressure. If the trousers are inflated to the point of pop-off valve activation and there has been no hemodynamic response in 30 minutes, the inflation pressure should be reduced as resuscitation continues.

C. Deflation

1. Before deflation:

   a. Insert one of two large-caliber intravenous catheters in a peripheral vein and re-establish blood volume.

   b. Monitor the patient's heart rate and rhythm.

    c. Assemble standby surgical and anesthesiology team.

    d. The patient can be taken to surgery or transported to a definitive-care center with the device inflated.

2. Deflate the trousers slowly while monitoring the patient's blood pressure.

    a. Stop deflation if the blood pressure falls 5 mmHg and hold at that point until additional fluids are given to return and maintain the patient's blood pressure.

    b. Always begin deflating the abdominal segment **first.**

    c. Should the patient's blood pressure suddenly fall, reinflate the trousers until more fluid can be given and/or the hemorrhage can be controlled surgically.

3. **Remember,** deflation of the trousers without the re-establishment of blood volume will result in profound shock, cardiac arrest, and death of the patient. **The greatest danger in the use of these garments is in their premature and inappropriate removal.**

D. Contraindications

1. Absolute: pulmonary edema and unstable myocardial dysfunction.

2. Caution: intrathoracic hemorrhage, ruptured diaphragm, and severe central nervous system injury.

Complications /Potential Adverse Effects of the PASG

The inflation of the pneumatic antishock garment to combat hypotension may be associated with ischemia, compartment syndrome, and tissue loss. Injuries to the lower extremities are at a greater risk. (See Chapter 3–Shock.)

Chapter 4:
Thoracic Trauma

Objectives:

Upon completion of this topic, the physician will be able to identify and explain the dangers of thoracic injuries and the principles of management.

Specifically, the physician will be able to:

A. Identify and manage the following **immediately** life-threatening chest injuries evidenced in the **primary survey:**

1. Airway obstruction
2. Tension pneumothorax
3. Open pneumothorax (sucking chest wound)
4. Massive hemothorax
5. Flail chest
6. Cardiac tamponade

B. Identify and initiate treatment of the following **potentially** life-threatening injuries assessed during the **secondary survey:**

1. Pulmonary contusion
2. Myocardial contusion
3. Aortic disruption
4. Traumatic diaphragmatic hernia
5. Tracheobronchial disruption
6. Esophageal disruption

C. Explain the purpose of, define the complications of, and demonstrate the ability to perform needle thoracentesis, chest tube insertion, and pericardiocentesis in a surgical skill practicum.

Chapter 4:
Thoracic
Trauma

American College of Surgeons

I. Introduction

A. Incidence

Chest injuries cause one out of four trauma deaths in this country. Many patients die after reaching the hospital. These deaths might be prevented by an understanding of pathophysiological factors that lead to prompt diagnosis and treatment.

Because most injuries occur at a distance from a medical center, the features of thoracic injuries that require early intervention and influence transport are very important. Less than 15% of these injuries require operation. The remaining 85% may be managed by simple procedures within the capabilities of any physician taking this course. Therefore, responsibility for the initial management of most chest-injury patients falls on the shoulders of the local physician and not on the thoracic surgeon at the major medical center.

B. Pathophysiology

Chest injury often leads to tissue hypoxia. The hypoxia may result from diminished blood volume, failure to ventilate the lungs, contusion of pulmonary tissue leading to ventilation/perfusion mismatch, or changes in the pressure relationships within the pleural space that lead to displacement of mediastinal structures and collapse of the lung. **Because hypoxia is the most compelling feature of chest injury, early interventions are designed to ensure that an adequate amount of oxygen is delivered to the portions of the lung capable of normal ventilation and perfusion.** The first and easiest therapy to initiate is the administration of oxygen, using a mask and bag reservoir capable of delivering an FIO_2 in excess of 0.85.

C. Treatment Approach

1. The physician's preconceived and prioritized plan of action is:

    a. Primary survey

    b. Resuscitation

    c. Secondary survey

    d. Definitive care

2. Examination is guided by a high index of suspicion for specific injuries.

3. Immediately life-threatening injuries are treated as simply and quickly as possible. Only then are the potentially life-threatening injuries definitively approached for diagnosis and treatment.

4. Most life-threatening thoracic injuries are treated with an appropriately placed chest tube or needle, based on clinical skill capabilities.

II. Primary Survey of Life-threatening Chest Trauma

A. Airway

1. Assess for airway patency and air exchange by listening for air movement at the patient's nose and mouth.

2. The patient should also be assessed for intercostal and supraclavicular muscle retractions. The signs of chest injury or impending hypoxia, which are particularly important and often subtle, include: 1) an increased rate of breathing, and 2) a change in the breathing pattern, especially toward progressively more shallow respirations. Cyanosis appears very late during the course of hypoxia in the trauma patient because of the skin ischemia that may result from redistribution of blood volume in shocky patients, because decreased hemoglobin may be present, and because an amount of unsaturated hemoglobin sufficient to produce cyanosis (5 grams/100 ml of blood) may not be present.

3. Assess the oropharynx for foreign body obstruction, particularly in the unconscious patient.

B. Breathing

Expose the patient's chest completely, and evaluate the breathing. Assess respiratory movement and quality of respiration by observing, palpating, and auscultating.

C. Circulation

1. Assess the patient's pulse for quality, rate, regularity, and presence of paradox. **Remember,** hypovolemic patients may not have peripheral pulses in the radial and the dorsalis pedis.

2. Assess the blood pressure for width of pulse pressure.

3. Observe and palpate the skin for color and temperature to assess the peripheral circulation.

4. Check to see if the neck veins are distended. **Remember,** neck veins may not be distended in hypovolemic patients with cardiac tamponade.

5. A cardiac monitor should be attached to the patient. Patients sustaining thoracic trauma—especially in the area of the sternum, or involving a rapid deceleration injury—are subject to myocardial contusion and/or coronary artery spasm, rendering them susceptible to dysrhythmias. Hypoxia and/or acidosis enhance this possibility. A common dysrhythmia is premature ventricular contraction which may require treatment with an immediate lidocaine bolus followed by a lidocaine drip. The term electromechanical dissociation (EMD) is used in this course as a manifestation of cardiac tamponade, tension pneumothorax, and/or profound hypovolemia. It may also indicate cardiac rupture.

D. Open Thoracotomy

Closed heart massage for cardiac arrest or electromechanical dissociation is ineffective for a hypovolemic patient. Assuming a surgeon is present, the procedure of a left anterior thoracotomy, cross-clamping of the descending thoracic aorta, pericardiotomy, and open chest massage in conjunction with intravascular volume restoration may be initiated. Appropriate candidates may include patients with exsanguinating penetrating injuries, and those sustaining blunt injury who arrive pulseless but with myocardial electrical activity.

III. Life-threatening Chest Injuries Identified in the Primary Survey

A. Airway Obstruction

Airway obstruction at the alveolar level is a potentially life-threatening injury that is assessed and managed during the secondary survey and definitive-care phases. Chapter 2 deals with the management of life-threatening situations of the upper airway.

B. Tension Pneumothorax

A tension pneumothorax develops when a "one-way valve" air leak occurs either from the lung or through the chest wall. Air is forced into the thoracic cavity without any means of escape, completely collapsing the affected lung. The mediastinum and trachea are displaced to the opposite side, interfering with venous return and compressing ventilation of the other lung.

The most common causes of tension pneumothorax are mechanical ventilation with positive end-expiratory pressure, spontaneous pneumothorax in which ruptured emphysematous bullae have failed to seal, and blunt chest trauma in which the parenchymal lung injury has failed to seal. Occasionally traumatic defects in the chest wall may cause a tension pneumothorax. There is a significant incidence of pneumothorax associated with subclavian catheter insertion.

Tension pneumothorax is a clinical rather than radiologic diagnosis. A tension pneumothorax is identified by tracheal deviation, respiratory distress, unilateral absence of breath sounds, distended neck veins, and cyanosis as a late manifestation. A tension pneumothorax initially may be confused with cardiac tamponade; however, tension pneumothorax is more common. Differentiation may be made by a hypertympanic percussion note over the ipsilateral chest.

Tension pneumothorax requires **immediate decompression** and is managed initially by rapidly inserting a needle into the second intercostal space in the midclavicular line of the affected hemithorax. This maneuver converts the injury to a pneumothorax. Aspirating with a syringe attached to a needle is helpful. The ability to aspirate air easily confirms the diagnosis. In the event of failure to aspirate air, withdraw the syringe and needle. (Note: The possibility of subsequent pneumothorax as a result of the needle stick now exists).

Repeated reassessment is necessary. If air is aspirated, disconnect the syringe, leaving the needle in place. Definitive treatment usually requires only the insertion of a chest tube into the fifth intercostal space (nipple level), anterior to the midaxillary line.

C. Open Pneumothorax

Penetrating injury to the thorax usually seals itself. However, large defects occasionally remain open, causing a "sucking chest wound." Equilibration between intrathoracic pressure and atmospheric pressure is immediate. If the opening in the chest wall is approximately two-thirds the diameter of the trachea, air passes preferentially through the chest defect with each respiratory effort, because air tends to follow the path of least resistance through the large chest-wall defect. Effective ventilation is thereby impaired, leading to hypoxia.

Manage an open pneumothorax by promptly closing the defect with a sterile occlusive dressing, large enough to overlap the wound's edges and taped securely on three sides. Taping the occlusive dressing on three sides provides a flutter-type valve effect. As the patient breathes in, the dressing is occlusively sucked over the wound, preventing air from entering. When the patient exhales, the open end of the dressing allows air to escape. Securely taping all edges of the dressing can cause air to accumulate in the thoracic cavity, resulting in a tension pneumothorax. Any occlusive dressing (plastic wrap, Vaseline gauze, etc) may be used as a stopgap so rapid assessment can continue. Place a chest tube in an area remote from the open wound. Definitive surgical closure of the defect is usually required.

D. Massive Hemothorax

Massive hemothorax, although rare, is dramatic in appearance. It occurs as a result of more than 1500 ml of blood lost into the chest cavity. It is most commonly caused by a penetrating wound that disrupts the systemic or pulmonary vessels. It may also be the result of blunt trauma. The blood loss is complicated by hypoxia. The neck veins may be flat secondary to severe hypovolemia, or may be distended because of the mechanical effects of a chest cavity full of blood. This condition is discovered when shock is associated with the absence of breath sounds and/or dullness to percussion on one side of the chest.

Massive hemothorax is initially managed by the simultaneous restoration of volume deficits and decompression of the chest cavity. Large-caliber intravenous lines and rapid crystalloid infusion are begun and type-specific blood is administered as soon as possible. If an auto-transfusion device is available, it may be used. A single chest tube (#38 French) is inserted at the nipple level, anterior to the midaxillary line, and rapid restoration of volume continues as decompression of the chest cavity is completed. Some patients require thoracotomy. This decision is based on the rate of continuing blood loss (200 ml/hour). The volume of blood that initially drains from the chest tube is not as important as the rate of continuing blood loss, and to indicate the amount of intravenous replacement required to resuscitate the patient. Similarly, the color of the blood (arterial or venous) is a poor indicator of the necessity for thoracotomy.

Penetrating anterior chest wounds medial to the nipple line and posterior wounds medial to the scapula should alert the physician to the possible need for thoracotomy, because of possible damage to the great vessels, hilar structures, and the heart, with the associated potential for cardiac tamponade. In addition, the surgeon at the definitive-care center must be told of the presence or absence of complete pleural space evacuation and re-expansion of the lung. Open thoracotomy is **not** indicated unless a surgeon is present.

E. Flail Chest

A flail chest occurs when a segment of the chest wall does not have bony continuity with the rest of the thoracic cage. This condition usually results from trauma associated with multiple rib fractures. The presence of a flail chest segment results in severe disruption of normal chest wall movement. If the injury to the underlying lung is sufficient, it may produce serious hypoxia. The major difficulty in flail chest stems from the injury to the underlying lung. Although chest wall instability leads to paradoxical motion of the chest wall with inspiration and expiration, this defect alone does not cause hypoxia. Associated pain and underlying lung injury, giving rise to loss of compliance, will contribute to the respiratory pattern defect and lead to hypoxia.

Flail chest may not be initially apparent because of splinting of the chest wall. The patient moves air poorly, and movement of the thorax is asymmetrical and uncoordinated. Palpation of abnormal respiratory motion and crepitus of rib or cartilage fractures aids diagnosis. A satisfactory chest roentgenogram may suggest multiple rib fractures, but may not show costochondral separation. Arterial blood gases, suggesting respiratory failure with hypoxia, may also aid in diagnosing a flail chest.

Initial therapy includes adequate ventilation, administration of humidified oxygen, and careful control of crystalloid intravenous solutions to prevent overhydration. The injured lung in a flail chest is sensitive to both under-resuscitation of shock, and fluid overload. Specific measures to optimize fluid measurement must be taken for the patient with flail chest.

The definitive treatment is to re-expand the lung and ensure oxygenation as completely as possible. Some patients can be managed without the use of a ventilator. However, prevention of hypoxia is of paramount importance for the trauma patient, and a short period of intubation and ventilation may be necessary until the diagnosis of the entire injury pattern is complete. A careful assessment of the respiratory rate, arterial oxygen tension, and an estimate of the work of breathing will indicate appropriate timing for intubation and ventilation. Not all patients with a flail chest require immediate endotracheal intubation. It is sometimes preferable to delay intubation until cervical spine roentgenograms have been obtained.

F. Cardiac Tamponade

Cardiac tamponade most commonly results from penetrating injuries. Blunt injury may also cause the pericardium to fill with blood from the heart or great vessels. The human pericardial sac is a fixed fibrous structure, and only a relatively small amount of blood is required to restrict cardiac activity and interfere with cardiac filling. Correspondingly, removal of small amounts of blood or fluid, often as little as 15 to 20 ml, by pericardiocentesis may have enormous beneficial effects for the critically ill patient.

The classic Beck's triad consists of venous pressure elevation, decline in arterial pressure, and muffled heart tones. However, muffled heart tones are difficult to assess in the noisy emergency department. Distended neck veins, caused by the elevated central venous pressure, may be absent due to hypovolemia. Pulsus paradoxus, a decrease in systolic pressure during inspiration in excess of 10 mmHg, may also be absent in some of the patients with cardiac tamponade. In addition, tension pneumothorax–particularly on the left side–may mimic cardiac tamponade. Kussmaul's sign (a rise in venous pressure with inspiration when breathing spontaneously) is a true paradoxical venous pressure abnormality associated with tamponade.

Pericardiocentesis is indicated for patients who do not respond to the usual measures of resuscitation for hemorrhagic shock and who have the potential for cardiac tamponade. Insertion of a central venous line by the percutaneous infraclavicular subclavian route may aid diagnosis. Life-saving pericardiocentesis should not be delayed for this diagnostic adjunct. For the patient who is unresponsive to resuscitation, a high index of suspicion is all that is necessary to initiate pericardiocentesis by the subxyphoid method.

Even though pericardial tamponade is strongly suspected, the initial administration of intravenous fluid will raise the venous pressure and improve cardiac output transiently while preparations are made for pericardiocentesis. Cardiac tamponade is then managed by prompt pericardiocentesis via the subxyphoid route. The use of a plastic-sheathed needle is preferable, but the urgent priority is to aspirate several milliliters of blood from the pericardial sac. Because of the self-sealing qualities of the myocardium, aspiration of pericardial blood alone may temporarily relieve symptoms. However, all patients with positive pericardiocentesis due to trauma will require open thoracotomy and inspection of the heart. Pericardial aspiration may not be diagnostic or therapeutic if the blood in the pericardial sac is clotted, which might be the case after rapid bleeding. Preparations for transfer to a definitive-care center are necessary for such patients. Open pericardiotomy may be life-saving but is indicated **only** when a qualified surgeon is available.

Once these injuries and other immediate life-threatening injuries have been stabilized, attention may be directed to the secondary survey and definitive-care phase of potential life-threatening thoracic injuries.

IV. Potentially Lethal Chest Injuries Identified in the Secondary Survey

The secondary survey requires further in-depth physical examination, an upright chest film if the patient's condition permits, arterial blood gases, and an electrocardiogram. In addition to lung expansion and the presence of fluid, the chest film should be examined for widening of the mediastinum, a shift of the midline, or loss of anatomic detail. Multiple rib fractures and fractures of the first and/or second rib(s) are evidence of severe force delivered to the chest and underlying tissues.

Six potentially lethal injuries are considered here.

1. Pulmonary contusion

2. Myocardial contusion

3. Aortic disruption

4. Traumatic diaphragmatic hernia

5. Tracheobronchial disruption

6. Esophageal disruption

Unlike life-threatening conditions, these injuries are not obvious on initial physical examination. Diagnosis requires a high index of suspicion. All are more often missed than diagnosed during the initial posttraumatic period. However, if these injuries are overlooked, mortality increases.

A. Pulmonary Contusion With or Without Flail Chest

Pulmonary contusion, almost indistinguishable from Adult Respiratory Distress Syndrome (ARDS), is the most common potentially lethal chest injury seen in North America. It is potentially lethal because the resulting respiratory failure develops over time rather than occurring instantaneously. The definitive management also proceeds with time and requires close monitoring.

Evidence now shows that some patients may be managed selectively without endotracheal intubation or the use of the adjunctive ventilator. Patients are intubated and ventilated in the first hour after injury, if they are hypoxic, as previously defined, or if they are to be transferred to another center, or cared for in a hospital where monitoring facilities are limited. Appropriate local specialists should agree on the method of treatment and at what facility the patient will receive optimal care. Some associated medical conditions that predispose to the need for early intubation include:

1. Pre-existing chronic pulmonary disease

2. Impaired level of consciousness

3. Abdominal injury resulting in ileus or the need for exploratory celiotomy

4. Skeletal injuries requiring immobilization

5. Renal failure

If the patient cannot maintain satisfactory oxygenation or has any of the above complicating features, intubation and mechanical ventilation should be considered.

B. Myocardial Contusion

Myocardial contusion, although difficult to diagnose, is another potentially lethal injury from blunt chest trauma. The patient's reported complaints of discomfort are often bypassed as being associated with chest wall contusion or fractures of the sternum and/or ribs. The diagnosis of myocardial contusion is established by abnormalities on the electrocardiogram, serial enzyme determinations, two-dimensional echocardiography, and associated history of injury. The electrocardiographic changes are variable, and may even indicate frank myocardial infarction. Multiple, premature ventricular contractions, unexplained sinus tachycardia, atrial fibrillation, bundle branch block (usually right), and ST segment changes are the most common electrocardiographic findings.

Patients with myocardial contusion are at risk for sudden dysrhythmias. They should be admitted to the critical care unit for close observation and cardiac monitoring.

C. Traumatic Aortic Rupture

Traumatic aortic rupture is the most common cause of sudden death after an automobile accident or a fall from a great height. Tears of the aorta and major pulmonary arteries, most of which result from blunt trauma, are fatal at the accident scene 90% of the time. For survivors, salvage is frequently possible, if aortic rupture is identified early.

Aortic rupture tends to occur at the ligamentum arteriosum of the aorta. Continuity maintained by an intact advential layer prevents immediate death. One-half of the surviving patients will die each day in the hospital if left untreated. Some blood may escape into the mediastinum, but one characteristic shared by all survivors is that this is a **contained** hematoma. Other than the initial pressure drop associated with the loss of 500 ml to 1000 ml of blood, hypotension responds to intravascular infusion. Persistent or recurrent hypotension is usually due to an unidentified bleeding site. Although free rupture of a transected aorta into the left chest does occur and causes hypotension, it is usually fatal unless the patient is operated on within a few minutes.

A high index of suspicion triggered by the radiologic findings, followed by arteriography, are the means of making the diagnosis. Angiography should be performed liberally because the findings of the chest roentgenogram, especially the supine view, are undependable. Approximately 10% of the aortograms will be positive for aortic rupture if liberal indications for using angiography are employed for all patients with widened mediastinum. Adjunctive radiologic signs, which may or may not be present, indicate the likelihood of major vascular injury in the chest. They include:

1. Widened mediastinum

2. Fractures of the first and second ribs

3. Obliteration of the aortic knob

4. Deviation of the trachea to the right

5. Presence of a pleural cap

6. Elevation and rightward shift of the right mainstem bronchus

7. Depression of the left mainstem bronchus

8. Obliteration of space between the pulmonary artery and the aorta

9. Deviation of the esophagus (nasogastric tube) to the right

False positives and false negatives occur with each radiographic sign. Therefore, no single finding reliably predicts or excludes significant injury. A widened mediastinum is the most consistent finding. Arteriography is considered the gold standard. A computed tomography scan may be less reliable, and even if it is positive, it does not always provide the surgeon with adequate preoperative information. It cannot be stressed too strongly that the slightest suspicion of aortic injury should be confirmed angiographically.

The usual treatment is either direct repair of the aorta or resection of the injured area and grafting. A qualified surgeon should treat such a patient.

D. Traumatic Diaphragmatic Hernia

A traumatic diaphragmatic hernia is more commonly diagnosed on the left side because of the appearance of the bowel or nasogastric tube in the chest. Blunt trauma produces large radial tears that lead to herniation. Penetrating trauma produces small perforations that often take some time, even years, to develop into diaphragmatic hernias.

These injuries are missed initially if the chest film is misinterpreted as showing an elevated left diaphragm, acute gastric dilatation, a loculated pneumohemothorax, or a subpulmonary hematoma. Thus, the diagnosis is not clearly identified on the initial roentgenogram or after the chest tube evacuation of the left hemothorax or pneumothorax. The diagnosis should be confirmed by contrast radiography. Occasionally, the sight of a nasogastric tube curled up in the left lower chest will eliminate the need for these special studies. The appearance of peritoneal lavage fluid in the chest tube drainage confirms the diagnosis.

E. Tracheobronchial Tree Injuries

1. Larynx

Fractures of the larynx are a rare injury and are indicated by the following triad:

a. Hoarseness

b. Subcutaneous emphysema

c. Palpable fracture crepitus

If the patient's airway is totally obstructed or the patient is in severe respiratory distress, an attempt at intubation is warranted. If intubation is unsuccessful, a tracheostomy (not surgical cricothyroidotomy) is indicated, followed by operative repair.

2. Trachea

Direct trauma to the trachea, including the larynx, can be either penetrating or blunt. Blunt injuries may be subtle, and history is all-important. Penetrating trauma is overt and requires immediate surgical repair. Penetrating injuries are often associated with esophageal, carotid artery, and jugular vein trauma. Penetrating injuries caused by missiles are often associated with extensive tissue destruction surrounding the area of penetration because of the blast effect.

Noisy breathing indicates partial airway obstruction that suddenly may become complete. Absence of breathing suggests that complete obstruction already exists. When the level of consciousness is depressed, detection of significant airway obstruction is more subtle. Observations of labored respiratory effort may be the only clue to airway obstruction and tracheobronchial injury. Endoscopic procedures aid diagnosis.

3. Bronchus

Injury to a major bronchus is an unusual and fatal injury that is frequently overlooked. The majority of such injuries result from blunt trauma and occur within one inch of the carina. Although the majority of patients with this injury die at the scene, those who reach the hospital alive have a 30% mortality, often due to associated injuries.

If suspicion of a bronchial injury exists, immediate surgical consultation is warranted. A patient with a bronchial injury frequently presents with hemoptysis, subcutaneous emphysema, or tension pneumothorax with a mediastinal shift. A pneumothorax associated with a persistent large air leak after tube thoracotomy suggests a bronchial injury. A second chest tube may be necessary to overcome a very large leak. Bronchoscopy confirms the diagnosis of the injury.

Treatment of tracheobronchial injuries may require only airway maintenance until the acute inflammatory and edema processes resolve. Major deviation or compression of the trachea by extrinsic masses, ie, hematomas, must be treated. Intubation frequently may be unsuccessful because of the anatomic distortion from paratracheal hematoma, major laryngotracheal injury, and associated injuries. For such patients, operative intervention is indicated. Patients surviving with bronchial injuries may require direct surgical intervention by thoracotomy.

F. Esophageal Trauma

Esophageal trauma is most commonly caused by penetrating trauma. Blunt esophageal trauma, although very rare, is lethal if unrecognized. Blunt injury of the esophagus is caused by a forceful injection of gastric contents into the esophagus from a severe blow to the upper abdomen. This forceful ejection produces a linear tear in the lower esophagus, allowing leakage into the mediastinum. The resulting mediastinitis and immediate or delayed rupture into the pleural space causes empyema. Other associated causes of esophageal trauma are primarily instrumentation.

The clinical picture is identical to that of postemetic esophageal rupture, so that diagnosis should be considered for any patient who has a left pneumothorax or hemothorax without a rib fracture; has received a severe blow to the lower sternum or epigastrium and is in pain or shock out of proportion to the apparent injury; or if particulate matter appears in the chest tube drainage after the blood begins to clear. The presence of mediastinal air, usually on the left side, is basis for diagnosis. The diagnosis can often be readily confirmed by gastrografin swallow and/or esophagoscopy.

Wide drainage of the pleural space and mediastinum with direct repair of the injury via thoracotomy is the treatment, if feasible. If the repair is tenuous or not feasible, esophageal diversion in the neck and gastrostomy of the lower and upper gastric segments usually is carried out, thereby avoiding continued soiling of the mediastinum and pleura by gastric and esophageal contents.

V. Other Manifestations of Chest Injuries

A. Subcutaneous Emphysema

Subcutaneous emphysema may result from airway injury; lung injury; or rarely, blast injury. It does not require treatment.

B. Crushing Injury to the Chest

Findings associated with a crush injury to the chest include subcutaneous emphysema; and upper torso, facial, and arm plethora with petechiae secondary to superior vena cava compression.

C. Simple Pneumothorax

Pneumothorax results from air entering the potential space between the visceral and parietal pleura. Both penetrating and nonpenetrating trauma may cause this injury. Lung laceration with air leakage is the most common cause of pneumothorax resulting from blunt trauma.

The thorax is normally completely filled by the lung, held to the chest wall by surface tension between the pleural surfaces. Air in the pleural space collapses lung tissue. This collapsed lung does not participate in oxygen exchange. A ventilation perfusion defect occurs because the blood circulated to the nonventilated area is not oxygenated.

When a pneumothorax is present, percussion of the chest shows hyperresonance. Breath sounds are usually decreased or absent. An expiratory roentgenogram of the chest may aid the diagnosis. If the injuries are so critical that obtaining a chest roentgenogram would jeopardize the patient's status, needle aspiration as described for a tension pneumothorax may establish the diagnosis.

A pneumothorax associated with other injuries is best treated with a chest tube in the fourth or fifth intercostal space, anterior to the midaxillary line. Observation and/or aspiration of any pneumothorax is risky. Once a chest tube has been inserted and connected to an underwater seal apparatus with 20 to 30 cm of water suction, a roentgenogram of the chest is necessary to confirm re-expansion of the lung. General anesthesia should never be administered for definitive care of injuries in patients who have sustained traumatic pneumothorax, or who are at risk for unexpected intraoperative pneumothorax, until a chest tube has been inserted. The chest should also be decompressed before transporting the patient with a pneumothorax via air ambulance.

D. Hemothorax

The primary cause of hemothorax is lung laceration, or laceration of an intercostal vessel or internal mammary artery due to either penetrating or blunt trauma. In the vast majority of cases this bleeding is self-limiting and does not require operative intervention.

Hemothorax, sufficient to appear on chest roentgenogram, is usually treated with a large-caliber chest tube. Intubation of the pleural space allows evacuation of blood and reduces the risk of clotted hemothorax, which may lead to pulmonary restriction, and subsequent thoracotomy and decortication. Intubation also provides a monitoring method. While many factors are involved in the decision to operate on a patient with a hemothorax, the amount of blood drainage from the chest tube is a major factor. If a liter of blood is obtained through the chest tube, surgical consultation is warranted. Persistent drainage of more than 200 ml per hour for four hours may indicate the need for thoracotomy.

E. Rib Fractures

The ribs are the most commonly injured component of the thoracic cage. Injuries to the ribs are often significant. Pain on motion results in splinting of the thorax, which impairs ventilation. Tracheobronchial secretions cannot be easily eliminated. The incidence of atelectasis and pneumonia rises strongly with pre-existing lung disease.

The upper ribs (1-3) are protected by the bony framework of the upper limb. The scapula, humerus, and clavicle, along with their muscular attachments, provide a barrier to injury in this area. Fractures of the first or second rib often indicate major injury to the head, neck, spinal cord, lungs, and the great vessels. Because of the severity of the associated injuries, mortality can be as high as 50%.

The middle ribs (4-9) sustain the majority of blunt trauma. Anteroposterior compression of the thoracic cage will bow the ribs outward with a fracture in the midshaft. Direct force applied to the ribs tends to fracture them and drive the ends of the bones into the thorax with more potential for intrathoracic injury, such as a pneumothorax. As a general rule, a young patient with a more flexible chest wall is less likely to sustain rib fractures. Therefore, the presence of multiple rib fractures in young patients implies a more sizable force transfer than in older patients.

Localized pain, tenderness on palpation, and crepitus are present in rib injury patients. A palpable or visible deformity suggests rib fractures. A roentgenogram of the chest should be obtained primarily to exclude other intrathoracic injuries and not just to identify rib fractures. Fractures of anterior cartilages or separation of costochondral junctions have the same implications as rib fractures but will not be seen on the roentgenographic examinations. Special rib technique roentgenograms are expensive, may not detect all rib injuries, add nothing to treatment, require painful positioning of the patient, and are not useful. Taping, rib belts, and external splints are contraindicated.

F. Other Indications for Chest Tube Insertion

1. In selected cases with suspected severe lung injury, especially those being transferred by air or ground vehicle.

2. Individuals undergoing general anesthesia for treatment of other injuries (eg, cranial or extremity), and individuals requiring positive pressure ventilation.

VI. Summary

Thoracic trauma is quite common in the multiply injured patient and can be associated with life-threatening problems. These problems can usually be relieved with simple measures such as tube thoracostomy or needle pericardiocentesis. The physician must possess the cognitive knowledge to diagnose these life-threatening thoracic injuries, and must develop the manipulative skills to perform the associated life-saving techniques. The specific details of tube thoracostomy and needle pericardiocentesis are presented in the skill station section. The high incidence of thoracic trauma also necessitates routine ECG monitoring of all multiply injured patients. This monitoring can be at times forgotten in the busy trauma room. A thorough understanding of thoracic injuries and their proper treatment can be rewarding for the physician and may save the patient's life.

Bibliography

1. Blair E, Topuzulu C, Deane RS: Major Chest Trauma. **Current Problems in Surgery** May 1969; pp 2-69.

2. Champion HR, Danne PD, Finelli F: Emergency Thoracotomy. **Archives of Emergency Medicine** 1986; 3:95-99.

3. Evans J, Gray LA Jr, Rayner A, et al: Principles for Management of Penetrating Cardiac Wounds. **Annals of Surgery** 1979; 189 (6):777-784.

4. Fulton FL: Penetrating Wounds of the Heart. **Heart and Lung** 1978; 7(2):262-268.

5. Graham JG, Mattox KL, Beall AC Jr: Penetrating Trauma of the Lung. **Journal of Trauma** 1979; 19:665.

6. Jones KW: Thoracic Trauma. **Surgical Clinics of North America** 1980; 60-957.

7. Kirsh MM, Behrendt DM, Orringer MB, et al: The Treatment of Acute Traumatic Rupture of the Aorta: a 10-year Experience. **Annals of Surgery** 1976; 184:308.

8. Liedtke AJ, DeMuth WE: Nonpenetrating Cardiac Injuries: A Collective Review. **American Heart Journal** 1973; 86:687.

9. Marnocha KE, Maglinte DDT, Woods J, et al: Blunt Chest Trauma and Suspected Aortic Rupture: Reliability of Chest Radiograph Findings. **Annals of Emergency Medicine** 1985; 14(7):644-649.

10. Mattox KL, Feliciano DV: Role of External Cardiac Compression in Truncal Trauma. **Journal of Trauma** 1982;22:934-936.

11. Mattox KL, Espada R, Beall AC, Jr; Performing Thoracotomy in the Emergen–cy Center. **Journal of the American College of Emergency Physicians** 1974; 3:13.

12. Mulder DS, Schennid H, Angood P: Thoracic Injuries, in Maull KI, Cleveland HC, Strauch GO, et al (ed):. **Trauma Volume 1**, Chicago, Yearbook, 1986.

13. Richardson JD, Adams L, Flint LM: Selective Management of Flail Chest and Pulmonary Contusion. **Annals of Surgery** 1982; 196(4):481-487.

14. Roberge RJ, Ivatury RR, Stahl W, et al: Emergency Department Thoracotomy for Penetrating Injuries: Predictive Value of Patient Classification. **American Journal of Emergency Medicine** 1986; 4(2):129-135.

15. Shannon FL, Moore EE, Moore JB: Emergency Department Thoracotomy, in Mattox KL, Moore EE, Feliciano DV (ed): **Trauma**, Appleton-Lange, 1988.

16. Snow N, Lucas AE, Richardson JD: Intra-aortic Balloon Counterpulsation for Cardiogenic Shock from Cardiac Contusion. **Journal of Trauma** 1982; 22(5): 426-429.

Chapter 4:
Thoracic
Trauma

Skill
Station
VII

Skill Station VII:
Chest Trauma Management

This surgical procedure, if performed on a live, anesthetized animal, must be conducted in a USDA Registered Animal Laboratory Facility. (See *ATLS Instructor Manual*, Section II, Chapter 10—Animal Laboratory Guidelines and Protocols.)

Equipment

1. Live, anesthetized animals
2. Licensed veterinarian (see guidelines reference above)
3. Animal troughs, ropes (sandbags optional)
4. Animal intubation equipment
   a. Endotracheal tubes
   b. Laryngoscope blade and handle
   c. Respirator with 15-mm adapter
5. Electric shears with #40 blade
6. Tables or instrument stands
7. Needles
   a. Assorted #14-gauge over-the-needle catheters (3 to 6 cm long)
   b. #18-gauge spinal needles (5 to 6 inches long)
   c. #22-gauge spinal needles (5 to 6 inches long)
8. Syringes
   a. 6-ml syringes
   b. 12- ml syringes
   c. 35-ml syringes, plastic and glass
9. Suture
   a. 2-0 and 3-0 silk with cutting needle
   b. 2-0 and 3-0 silk with taper needle
   c. 4-0 Monofilament/noncutting needle (optional)
10. Drugs
    a. Lidocaine 1% (optional)
    b. Heparin 1:1000 (optional)
11. Chest tubes–#32 French (for animal use); #36-40 French (for patient use)
12. 3x3s or 4x4s
13. One-inch adhesive tape
14. Underwater seal bottle or device
15. Small basin for water to inject into pericardial sac (methylene-blue dye may be added to the water for a more dramatic appearance when performing the pericardiocentesis)
16. Flutter-type valve

Chapter 4:
Thoracic
Trauma

Skill
Station
VII

17. Stopcocks–three-way

18. Surgical instruments

    a. Scalpel handles with #10 and #11 blades

    b. Needle holders

    c. Small Finochetti chest retractors or small self-retaining chest retractors

    d. Mosquitoes

    e. Heavy curved scissors

    f. Suture scissors

    g. Metsenbaum curved dissecting scissors

    h. Tissue forceps–with and without teeth

19. Antiseptic swabs

20. Surgical drapes (optional)

21. Electrocardiographic monitor (optional)

22. Surgical garb (gloves, shoe covers, and scrub suits or cover gowns)

Objectives

1. Performance at this station will allow the participant to practice and demonstrate on a live, anesthetized animal the techniques of inserting a chest needle, and chest tube for the emergency care of hemothoraces and/or pneumothoraces.

2. Upon completion of this station, the participant will be able to describe the surface markings and technique for pleural decompression with needle thoracentesis and chest tube insertion.

3. Upon completion of this station, the participant will be able to discuss the underlying pathophysiology of cardiac tamponade as a result of trauma.

4. Upon completion of this station, the participant will be able to describe the surface markings and technique for pericardiocentesis.

5. Performance at this station will allow the participant to practice and demonstrate on a live, anesthetized animal the technique of inserting a needle into the pericardium (pericardiocentesis) for the emergency treatment of cardiac tamponade or hemopericardium.

6. Upon completion of this station, the participant will be able to discuss the complications of needle thoracentesis, chest tube insertion, and pericardiocentesis.

Procedures

1. Needle thoracentesis

2. Chest tube insertion

3. Pericardiocentesis

Chapter 4:
Thoracic
Trauma

Skill
Station
VII

Skills Procedures

Chest Trauma Management

I. Needle Thoracentesis

Note: This procedure is for the rapidly deteriorating critical patient who has a life-threatening tension pneumothorax. If this technique is used and the patient does not have a tension pneumothorax, there is a 10% to 20% risk of producing a pneumothorax and/or causing damage to the lung.

A. Assess the patient's chest and respiratory status.

B. Apply oxygen at 12 liters per mask, or administer oxygen under positive pressure with a bag-valve-mask device.

C. Identify the second intercostal space, in the midclavicular line on the side of the pneumothorax.

D. Surgically prepare the chest.

E. Locally anesthetize the area if the patient is conscious or if time permits.

F. Attach an over-the-needle catheter (3 to 6 cm long) very snugly to a 35-ml syringe.

G. Place the patient in an upright position if a cervical spine injury has been ruled out.

H. Insert the needle into the skin and direct the needle just over (ie, superior to) the rib into the intercostal space.

I. Puncture the parietal pleura.

J. Aspirate as much air as necessary to relieve the patient's acute symptoms.

K. Leave the plastic catheter in place and apply a bandage or small dressing.

L. Prepare for a chest-tube insertion, if necessary. The chest tube should be inserted at the nipple level anterior to the midaxillary line of the affected hemithorax.

M. Connect the chest tube to an underwater seal device or a flutter-type valve apparatus.

N. Obtain a chest roentgenogram.

Complications of Needle Thoracentesis

1. Local cellulitis
2. Local hematoma
3. Pleural infection, empyema
4. Pneumothorax

**Chapter 4:
Thoracic
Trauma**

**Skill
Station
VII**

II. Chest Tube Insertion

A. Fluid resuscitation via at least one, large-caliber intravenous catheter, and monitoring of vital signs should be in process.

B. Determine the insertion site: usually the nipple level (5th intercostal space) anterior to the midaxillary line on the affected side. A second chest tube may be used for a hemothorax.

C. Prep and drape the chest at the predetermined site of the tube insertion.

D. Locally anesthetize the skin and rib periosteum.

E. Make a 2- to 3-cm transverse (horizontal) incision at the predetermined site and bluntly dissect through the subcutaneous tissues, just over the top of the rib.

F. Puncture the parietal pleura with the tip of a clamp and put a gloved finger into the incision to avoid injury to other organs, and to clear any adhesions, clots, etc.

G. Clamp the proximal end of the thoracostomy tube and advance the thoracostomy tube into the pleural space to the desired length.

H. Look for "fogging" of the chest tube with expiration or listen for air movement.

I. Connect the end of the thoracostomy tube to an underwater-seal apparatus.

J. Suture the tube in place.

K. Apply a dressing, and tape the tube to the chest.

L. Obtain a chest roentgenogram.

M. Obtain arterial blood gases as necessary.

Complications of Chest Tube Insertion

1. Anaphylactic or allergic reaction to surgical prep or anesthetic
2. Chest tube dislodgment from the chest wall or disconnection from the underwater-seal apparatus
3. Chest bottle elevated above the level of the chest, and fluid flows into the chest cavity
4. Chest tube kinking or clogging
5. Damage to the intercostal nerve, artery, or vein
   a. converting a pneumothorax to a hemopneumothorax
   b. resulting in intercostal neuritis/neuralgia
6. Damage to internal mammary vessels if puncture is too medial, resulting in hemopneumothorax
7. Incorrect tube position, extra- or intrathoracically
8. Intercostal myalgia
9. Introduction of pleural infection (eg, thoracic empyema)

Chapter 4:
Thoracic
Trauma

Skill
Station
VII

10. Laceration or puncture of intrathoracic and/or abdominal organs, all of which can be prevented by using the finger technique before inserting the chest tube.
    a. Heart
    b. Lung
    c. Esophagus
    d. Aorta
    e. Pulmonary artery
    f. Pulmonary vein
    g. Long thoracic nerve
    h. Mediastinum
    i. Liver
    j. Spleen
11. Leaky underwater-seal apparatus
12. Local cellulitis
13. Local hematoma
14. Mediastinal emphysema
15. Persistent pneumothorax
    a. Large primary leak
    b. Leak at the skin around the chest tube; suction on tube too strong
    c. Leaky underwater-seal apparatus
16. Subcutaneous emphysema (usually at tube site)
17. Recurrence of pneumothorax upon removal of chest tube; seal of thoracostomy wound not immediate
18. Lung fails to expand due to plugged bronchus; bronchoscopy required

III. Pericardiocentesis

A. Monitor the patient's vital signs, central venous pressure, and electrocardiogram before, during, and after the procedure.

B. Prepare the xiphoid and subxiphoid areas, if time allows.

C. Locally anesthetize the puncture site, if necessary.

D. Using a #16- to #18-gauge, 6-inch or longer over-the-needle catheter, attach a 35 ml empty syringe with a three-way stopcock.

E. Assess the patient for any mediastinal shift that may have caused the heart to shift significantly.

F. Puncture the skin 1 to 2 cm inferior to the left of the xiphochondral junction, at a 45-degree angle to the skin.

G. Carefully advance the needle cephalad and aim toward the tip of the left scapula.

H. If the needle is advanced too far (into the ventricular muscle) an injury pattern (eg, extreme ST-T wave changes, or widened and enlarged QRS complex) will appear on the electrocardiogram monitor. This pattern indicates that the pericardiocentesis needle should be withdrawn until the previous baseline electrocardiogram tracing reappears. Premature ventricular contractions may also occur, secondary to irritation of the ventricular myocardium.

**Chapter 4:
Thoracic
Trauma**

**Skill
Station
VII**

I. When the needle tip enters the blood-filled pericardial sac, withdraw as much nonclotted blood as possible.

J. During the aspiration, the epicardium will reapproach the inner pericardial surface, as will the needle tip. Subsequently, an electrocardiogram injury pattern may reappear. This indicates that the pericardiocentesis needle should be withdrawn slightly. Should this injury pattern persist, withdraw the needle completely.

K. After aspiration is completed, remove the syringe, and attach a three-way stopcock, leaving the stopcock closed. Secure the catheter in place.

L. Should the cardiac tamponade symptoms persist, the stopcock may be opened and the pericardial sac reaspirated. The plastic pericardiocentesis needle can be sutured or taped in place, and covered with a small dressing to allow for continued decompression en route to surgery or transfer to another care facility.

Complications of Pericardiocentesis

1. Aspiration of left or right ventricular cavity blood instead of pericardial blood
2. Cellulitis
3. Laceration of coronary artery or vein
4. Laceration of ventricular epicardium/myocardium
5. New hemopericardium, secondary to lacerations of the coronary artery or vein,   and/or ventricular epicardium/myocardium
6. Local hematoma
7. Pericarditis
8. Ventricular fibrillation, secondary to microcurrent leak
9. Pneumothorax, secondary to lung puncture
10. Puncture of aorta
11. Puncture of inferior vena cava
12. Puncture of esophagus
13. Mediastinitis secondary to puncture of esophagus
14. Puncture of peritoneum
15. Peritonitis, secondary to puncture of peritoneum

Chapter 5:
Abdominal Trauma

Objectives:

Upon completion of this topic, the physician will be able to identify the differences in the patterns of abdominal trauma based on injury mechanism, and establish management priorities accordingly. Specifically, the physician will be able to:

A. Describe the anatomic regions of the abdomen.

B. Discuss the difference in injury pattern between blunt and penetrating trauma.

C. Identify the signs suggesting retroperitoneal, intraperitoneal, or pelvic injury.

D. Outline the diagnostic and therapeutic procedures specific to abdominal trauma.

E. Define the indications, technique, interpretation, and complications of diagnostic peritoneal lavage; and demonstrate the ability to perform this procedure on a live, anesthetized animal.

Chapter 5:
Abdominal
Trauma

American College of Surgeons

I. Introduction

A. High Index of Suspicion

Unrecognized abdominal injury remains a distressingly frequent cause of preventable death after trauma. Peritoneal signs are often subtle, overshadowed by pain from associated extra-abdominal trauma or masked by head injury or intoxicants. As many as 20% of patients with acute hemoperitoneum will have a benign abdominal examination when first examined in the emergency department. Moreover, the peritoneal cavity is a potential reservoir for major occult blood loss. Any patient sustaining significant deceleration injury or a penetrating torso wound must be assumed to have an abdominal visceral injury.

The primary factor in assessing and managing abdominal trauma is not the accurate diagnosis of a specific type of injury, but rather the determination that an intra-abdominal injury exists and operative intervention is required.

B. Blunt Versus Penetrating

The abdominal injury pattern of blunt trauma is much different from that of penetrating wounds. Blunt vehicular trauma results from rapid changes in speed in which visceral disruption may occur from a direct blow, shear forces, or closed-loop phenomenon. The liver, spleen, and kidney are the organs predominantly involved following blunt trauma, although the relative incidence of hollow visceral perforation and lumbar spinal injuries increases with incorrect seat belt usage.

The injuries produced by penetration may involve indirect effects, such as blast or cavitation, as well as the injury incurred as a result of the anatomic course of the weapon or object inflicting the wound. The injury pattern correlates with the relative size of the abdominal viscera and their proximity to the entrance site. As expected, liver, small bowel, colon, and stomach are commonly involved. Stab injuries traverse adjacent structures, whereas gunshot wounds may have a circuitous trajectory, injuring multiple noncontiguous organs.

C. Regions of the Abdomen

The abdomen has three distinct anatomic compartments—peritoneum, retroperitoneum, and pelvis.

The **peritoneal cavity** may be further divided into intrathoracic and abdominal segments. The **intrathoracic abdomen** is that portion covered by the bony thorax, and includes the diaphragm, liver, spleen, stomach, and transverse colon. The diaphragm may rise to the fourth intercostal space with full expiration, rendering the viscera at risk after lower chest trauma—particularly penetrating wounds. Fractures of the lower ribs should increase suspicion for hepatosplenic injury.

The **retroperitoneum** contains the aorta, vena cava, pancreas, kidneys, and ureters, and portions of the colon and duodenum. Injuries to the retroperitoneal viscera are notoriously difficult to recognize because the area is remote from physical examination and not sampled by peritoneal lavage.

The pelvis houses the rectum; bladder; iliac vessels; and in women, the internal genitalia. Early diagnosis of trauma to these structures is similarly compromised because of anatomic location.

II. History

A. Blunt Trauma

Details of the accident are particularly helpful in the initial evaluation of blunt multisystem trauma. This critical information should be obtained directly from the prehospital personnel before they leave the emergency department. Important questions include time of injury, mechanism and estimated speed of impact, damage to involved vehicles, use and type of restraining devices, and condition of other accident victims.

B. Penetrating Wounds

Valuable facts in the assessment of penetrating injuries include time of injury, type of weapon (ie, knife length), handgun caliber (ie, muzzle velocity), distance from assailant (particularly for shotgun wounds), number of stab attempts or shots taken, and amount of blood at the scene. The patient, if conscious, is best prepared to provide most of this information, but police may also glean this data from their preliminary investigation.

III. Physical Examination

A positive physical examination is the most reliable clinical sign of significant intra-abdominal trauma. Conversely a negative physical examination does not preclude significant intra-abdominal injury. Unequivocal signs of peritoneal irritation–involuntary muscle guarding, diffuse or rebound tenderness–warrant expeditious celiotomy without additional confirmatory tests.

The abdominal examination should be conducted in a meticulous, systematic fashion in the standard sequence; ie, inspection, auscultation, percussion, and palpation. These findings, whether positive or negative, should be documented carefully in the medical records. For many patients, initial abdominal assessment is rendered inadequate due to the confounding factors discussed above, and telltale signs of visceral injury become apparent only on follow-up examination.

A. Inspection

The patient must be fully undressed. The anterior and posterior abdomen as well as lower chest should be inspected for abrasions, contusions, lacerations, and penetrating wounds. The patient must be log-rolled to facilitate complete examination; the back and perineum are most frequently overlooked.

B. Auscultation

The abdomen should be auscultated for the presence or absence of bowel sounds. Free intraperitoneal blood or enteric contents may produce ileus, resulting in loss of bowel sounds. Ileus, however, may also occur from extra-abdominal injuries; ie, rib, spine, and pelvic fractures. A bruit heard after a penetrating wound suggests a major arteriovenous fistula.

C. Percussion

Percussion of the abdomen after injury is done primarily to elicit subtle rebound tenderness. This maneuver generates slight motion of the peritoneum, and produces a similar response to asking the patient to cough.

D. Palpation

Palpation of the abdomen results in subjective as well as objective information. Subjective findings include the patient's assessment of pain location as well as magnitude. Early pain is usually visceral in origin and, therefore, poorly localized. Voluntary tensing of the abdominal musculature results from the fear of pain and may not represent significant injury. Involuntary muscle guarding, on the other hand, is a reliable sign of peritoneal irritation. Similarly, unequivocal rebound tenderness indicates established peritonitis.

E. Rectal Examination

Digital rectal examination is an important component of the abdominal assessment. Major assessment goals for penetrating wounds are to search for blood, indicating bowel perforation, and ascertain sphincter tone to assess spinal integrity. After blunt trauma, the rectal wall should also be palpated for fractured bony elements and prostate position related to urethral disruption.

F. Vaginal Examination

Laceration of the vagina may occur from penetrating wounds or bony fragments from pelvic fracture. The implications of vaginal bleeding in the pregnant patient are reviewed in Chapter 11.

IV. Initial Management

Resuscitation and management priorities of the patient with major abdominal trauma follow the sequence detailed in Chapter 1.

A–Airway maintenance with c-spine control
B–Breathing
C–Circulation with hemorrhage control

Specific treatment of abdominal injuries should not supersede these critical measures to optimize oxygen delivery and tissue perfusion.

A. Blood Sampling

Blood should be withdrawn from one of the initial venous access catheters and sent to the laboratory for immediate analysis. Laboratory screening for suspected abdominal trauma includes a hematocrit, white blood count with differential, and amylase determination. These baseline tests are important, because subsequent changes may be the first sign of occult injury, particularly in the retroperitoneum. Blood type and crossmatching should be additionally requested for the severely injured patient.

B. Nasogastric Tube

Nasogastric intubation is both therapeutic and diagnostic. The primary goal is to remove stomach contents, reducing gastric volume and pressure, and thus, the risk for gastric aspiration. The presence of blood in stomach secretions suggests upper gastrointestinal disruption.

Caution: The gastric tube should be introduced via the mouth if a severe maxillary fracture exists. A nasogastric tube can be introduced into the cranium when a cribriform plate fracture exists.

C. Bladder Catheter

The indwelling urinary catheter serves dual purposes. The major function is to decompress the bladder and allow for urinary output monitoring as an index of circulatory perfusion. Hematuria is an important sign of potential genitourinary trauma; the implications are discussed later in this chapter.

Caution: A rectal examination should be performed before the urinary catheter is inserted if a pelvic fracture is suspected. A high-riding prostate, blood at the urethral meatus, or scrotal hematoma is a contraindication for placing an indwelling bladder catheter. In these situations, and if the bladder can be palpated, a percutaneous suprapubic cystostomy deserves consideration. A surgeon should perform such a procedure.

D. Screening Roentgenographs

Roentgenographic studies must be tailored to the patient's overall status as well as injury mechanism. The crosstable lateral cervical spine, chest, and pelvis films take precedence in multisystem blunt trauma. Free air under the diaphragm or extraluminal air in the retroperitoneum signals hollow visceral disruption, and mandates prompt celiotomy.

V. Indications for Early Surgical Intervention

Physical evidence of abdominal trauma in the hemodynamically unstable patient mandates immediate celiotomy. As mentioned previously, further unequivocal signs of peritoneal irritation warrant early abdominal exploration. Unfortunately, most patients requiring emergent operation for visceral injury do not manifest these obvious indications when first examined in the emergency department. Moreover, the abdominal examination may appear significant due to local abdominal wall injury or referred pain and secondary muscle spasm from rib, spine, or pelvis fractures. A broad-spectrum antibiotic should be administered in the emergency department after the decision for celiotomy has been made.

A. Blunt Trauma

1. Diagnostic peritoneal lavage

The necessity for emergent celiotomy in the multisystem blunt trauma patient is often difficult to establish, and must be sequenced properly among other potentially life-saving procedures. For these reasons, diagnostic peritoneal lavage (DPL) is a critical step in the evaluation of blunt trauma. For children, computed tomography scanning is often used in place of diagnostic peritoneal lavage. The only absolute contraindication to the procedure is an existing indication for celiotomy. Relative contraindications include previous abdominal operations, morbid obesity, advanced cirrhosis, established pre-existing coagulopathy, and advanced pregnancy.

Caution: Peritoneal lavage is an operative procedure and significantly alters subsequent examination of the patient. Therefore, the procedure should be performed by the surgeon caring for the patient. If a positive diagnostic peritoneal lavage will result in the patient's transfer, the procedure should be done by the referring physician. Any lavage fluid obtained should be sent with the patient. Diagnostic peritoneal lavage has a small but real incidence of technical complications, and should only be performed by experienced personnel.

a. Peritoneal lavage should be done for the multiply injured patient if the abdominal examination is:

1) **Equivocal** (fractured lower ribs, and pelvic and lumbar spine fractures may obscure findings).

2) **Unreliable** due to head injury, intoxicants, or paraplegia.

3) **Impractical** because of anticipated lengthy roentgenographic studies (angiography), or general anesthesia for extra-abdominal injuries.

b. Peritoneal lavage is also indicated if there is unexplained hypotension or blood loss (decreased hematocrit).

c. Peritoneal aspirate and lavage criteria indicating the need for emergent celiotomy are:

1) Aspiration of peritoneal cavity

a) > 5 ml gross blood

b) obvious enteric contents

Caution: Catheter aspiration of the normal uninjured peritoneal cavity may yield up to 5 ml of clear fluid.

2) Peritoneal lavage fluid is observed to exit via:

a) Chest tube—diaphragm injury (Failure to recover the DPL fluid should raise concern that the fluid has entered the thorax via a diaphragmatic tear.)

b) Indwelling urinary catheter (bladder perforation)

3) Laboratory analysis of peritoneal lavage fluid

   a) $> 100,000$ red blood cells/mm^3

   b) > 500 white blood cells/mm^3

   c) Amylase > 175 international units. (This is now controversial. There is serious question of its cost and benefit.)

   d)   Rarely does the presence of bacteria, vegetable fibers, or an amylase $>$ than serum levels constitute the sole criterion for celiotomy. However, when they occur they indicate intra-abdominal injury.

Peritoneal lavage findings are falsely negative in 2% of cases; ie, findings do not reflect evidence of significant intra-abdominal injury by standard criteria in one out of 50 to 100 patients. The false negative results are usually due to isolated injury of the: 1) pancreas, 2) duodenum, 3) diaphragm, 4) small bowel, or 5) bladder. The pancreas and duodenum are retroperitoneal structures and thus, are not sampled by diagnostic peritoneal lavage; injury to the latter three organs may be missed because they do not bleed sufficiently to produce $> 100,000$ RBCs/mm^3.

2. Adjunctive tests

Adjunctive tests, such as computed tomography of the abdomen and contrast studies of the urinary and gastrointestinal tracts, identify injuries that diagnostic peritoneal lavage misses.

Caution: Computed tomography (CT) of the abdomen has been suggested as a substitute for diagnostic peritoneal lavage for evaluation of isolated abdominal trauma in the stable patient. Diagnostic peritoneal lavage has been criticized as oversensitive in this situation, necessitating celiotomy due to RBC analysis for patients with minor liver trauma. While nonoperative management of these known types of injuries may be rational in an experienced Level I trauma center, it is not generally recommended to replace diagnostic peritoneal lavage because of the danger of delaying celiotomy. Moreover, several clinical studies have demonstrated that double-contrast computed tomography scanning may miss life-threatening intra-abdominal injuries.

a. Diaphragm

Blunt tears may occur in any portion of the diaphragm, including through the pericardium. The most common injury is 5 to 10 cm in length, involving the posterolateral left hemidiaphragm. Abnormalities on the initial chest roentgenogram are usually nonspecific. The position of the nasogastric tube may identify an otherwise occult left-sided tear; a coiled tube above the diaphragm is pathognomonic.

b. Duodenum

Duodenal rupture is classically encountered in the intoxicated, unrestrained driver involved in a frontal-impact motor vehicular accident. A bloody nasogastric aspirate should raise the suspicion of the physician. Duodenal "C-loop" gastrografin studies or double contrast computed tomography scanning is indicated for the high-risk patient following completion of the secondary survey.

c. Pancreas

Pancreatic fracture most often results from a direct epigastric blow compressing the organ against the vertebral column. Normal serum amylase does not exclude major pancreatic trauma; conversely, the amylase may be elevated from nonpancreatic sources. (Isoenzymes do not assist in differentiating.) Double contrast computed tomography scanning may not identify significant pancreatic trauma in the immediate post-injury period.

B. Penetrating Trauma

Decision-making in the management of penetrating abdominal injury is relatively simple compared to blunt trauma. Overt signs of peritoneal irritation or acute blood loss remain unquestionable indications for immediate celiotomy. However, initial physical examination is frequently misleading, yielding false positive results in 10% to 15% and false negative in 20% to 35%. An aggressive policy for abdominal exploration is justified because of the relatively high incidence of hollow visceral injury as well as major vascular involvement.

1. Gunshot wounds

Gunshot wounds to the abdomen mandate celiotomy if the missile has entered the peritoneum; 95% of such explorations will disclose significant visceral injury. If an exit wound is not evident, plain roentgenographic studies are critical to determine missile trajectory. Broad-spectrum antibiotics should be routinely administered to patients sustaining a gunshot wound to the abdomen.

2. Stab wounds

Stab wounds to the abdomen pose a lesser risk for serious visceral injury compared to gunshot wounds, but are equally difficult to assess by physical examination. Most urban Level I trauma centers follow a selective celiotomy policy, because less than one-half of these patients require an emergent operation. Selectivity is usually based on sequential local wound exploration and peritoneal lavage. But unless the physician has substantial patient experience, the safest approach is to perform exploratory celiotomy for all suspected penetrating wounds. A patient with a presumed superficial wound may be observed if local wound exploration by a surgeon confirms that the underlying fascia is intact.

3. Lower chest wounds

The lower chest is defined as the area between the fourth intercostal space anteriorly (nipple line), the seventh intercostal space posteriorly (scapular tip), and the costal margins. Because the diaphragm rises to the fourth intercostal space during full expiration, penetrating wounds to this region may involve the underlying abdominal viscera. The incidence of significant organ injury with such an entrance site is 15% to 25% following a stab wound and 45% to 60% after a gunshot wound. The safest policy is routine celiotomy for lower chest gunshot wounds, while stab wounds can probably be managed more selectively.

4. Flank and back wounds

Penetrating injuries in the retroperitoneum are particularly difficult to evaluate because of their secluded anatomic location. An overlooked colon perforation can be fatal. The risk of significant visceral injury is 5% to 15% following back penetration and 20% to 30% from flank wounds.

Routine celiotomy, however, is the safest policy because there are no reliable tests to evaluate the retroperitoneum.

VI. Genitourinary Tract Injuries

Genitourinary trauma must be considered for all patients sustaining: 1) blunt deceleration trauma, or 2) penetrating abdominal wounds that enter the retroperitoneum or pelvis. Genitourinary injuries may occur without hematuria; the presence of blood in the urine after injury mandates urologic investigation. **Caution: Time-consuming urological studies should not be performed at the initial hospital if the patient is to be transferred to another facility.**

A. Blunt Trauma

Direct blows to the back or flank resulting in contusions, hematomas, or ecchymosis are markers of potential underlying renal injury. Fractures of posterior lower ribs or spinal transverse processes increase this probability. Similarly, perineal hematomas and anterior pelvic fractures suggest bladder or urethral trauma. Blood at the urethral meatus or the inability to void are overt signs of lower urinary tract injury. Urethral disruptions are divided into those above the urogenital diaphragm (posterior) or below (anterior). Posterior urethral trauma usually occurs in patients with multisystem injuries and pelvic fracture(s). Anterior urethral injury is due to a straddle impact, and is usually an isolated injury. Blunt renal artery thrombosis is infrequent, and renal pedicle disruption is rare; both lesions may not produce hematuria.

B. Penetrating Trauma

Penetrating wounds, particularly gunshot(s), to the back, flank, or pelvis may produce occult urologic injury. Some perforations of the ureter and bladder will not exhibit hematuria.

C. Roentgenographic Studies

1. Excretory urogram

Intravenous pyelography (IVP) remains a valuable initial renal evaluation. High-dose intravenous bolus injection (1 ml/lb up to 100 ml of 30% organic iodine solution) should provide evidence of relative kidney function at 5 to 10 minutes. Unilateral nonfunction implies massive parenchymal shattering or vascular pedicle interruption, but may be due to an absent kidney; nonfunction warrants urgent surgical consultation. Delayed films, supplemented with tomography, may be needed to further evaluate renal parenchyma as well as ureters.

2. Cystography

Bladder rupture is established with a gravity flow cystogram. A bulb syringe attached to the indwelling bladder catheter is held 15 cm above the patient, and 250 ml of water-soluble contrast is allowed to flow into the bladder. Anteroposterior, oblique, and postdrainage views are essential to definitively exclude injury. The order of IVP versus cystography is governed by index of suspicion for upper versus lower tract injury.

3. Computed tomography scan

Complex injuries may require additional contrast computed tomography scanning.

D. Urethrography

Urethrography should be performed before inserting an indwelling urinary catheter if a urethral tear is suspected. The urethrogram can be performed with a #12 French urinary catheter secured in the meatal fossa by balloon inflation to 3 ml. Undiluted contrast material is instilled with gentle pressure.

VII. Hemorrhage From Pelvic Fractures and Associated Injuries

Major hemorrhage from pelvic fractures is an extremely difficult management problem. The large bones of the pelvis have a generous blood supply, and the exposed bone bleeds briskly. The major muscle groups surrounding these bones are also very vascular. Numerous large veins attend the pelvis and are at high risk for disruption. Major arterial injury from pelvic trauma can lead to exsanguinating hemorrhage.

Mortality rates from open pelvic fracture exceed 50%. Most severe pelvic injuries result from auto-pedestrian, motorcycle, or high fall accidents.

Physical examination should include careful inspection of the perineum for ecchymosis or open wounds and systematic compression of the bony pelvis. Rectal and genitourinary injuries must be suspected for all patients with pelvic fractures. Major hemorrhage is usually associated with major pelvic disruption. However, single roentgenographic views of the pelvis may not reflect the extent of these fractures, particularly of the posterior elements.

Initial management priorities in pelvic fracture bleeding include adequate volume replacement, careful hemodynamic monitoring, and complete patient evaluation to exclude extrapelvic sources of blood loss. Peritoneal lavage should be performed at or above the umbilical ring to avoid the hematoma that frequently extends from the pelvis into the lower anterior abdominal wall. A negative lavage reliably excludes serious intraperitoneal bleeding. On the other hand, a positive lavage by RBC count must be interpreted cautiously. Approximately 15% of these patients will exhibit a false positive result, because the pelvic hematoma leaks into the free peritoneal cavity.

The pneumatic antishock garment (PASG) should be applied if there is hemodynamic instability. The device compresses the bony fragments and tamponades the associated venous bleeding. Patients stabilized hemodynamically with this approach should then be evaluated for external skeletal fixation. The patient who continues to bleed despite the PASG requires a critical triage decision. In the unstable individual with a grossly positive peritoneal aspirate, celiotomy is obligatory to treat potentially life-threatening intra-abdominal hemorrhage. On the other hand, if the patient with a positive lavage by RBC count is stabilized, prompt arteriography should be considered. Most persistent pelvic bleeding comes from small-caliber branches of the internal iliac artery that are amenable to percutaneous embolization. Arteriography will delineate the source of pelvic hemorrhage as well as possibly exclude additional intra-abdominal sites of continued blood loss.

VIII.Summary

Two major types of abdominal trauma occur: penetrating and blunt. **In either case, early evaluation by a surgeon is essential.**

A. Penetrating Trauma

A surgeon must evaluate all penetrating injuries of the abdomen. Penetrating trauma to the flanks, buttocks, and lower chest may produce intra-abdominal injuries as well and should be regarded with a high degree of suspicion.

B. Blunt Trauma

Intra-abdominal visceral damage must be strongly suspected following blunt trauma to the abdomen, especially because evidence is frequently subtle and misleading. Diagnosis of such injuries is often difficult, and an aggressive approach is mandatory. Multiple injuries are common, and common signs and symptoms guide diagnosis. If these are absent or obscured by other injuries, special techniques must be applied. Peritoneal lavage, properly performed, is a valuable diagnostic tool for these patients. A specific organ injury diagnosis is not necessary— only the finding of an acute abdominal injury.

C. Management

Management of penetrating and blunt trauma to the abdomen includes:

1. Re-establishing vital functions and optimizing oxygenation and tissue perfusion.

2. Delineating injury mechanism.

3. Maintaining a high index of suspicion related to occult vascular and retroperitoneal injuries.

4. Repeating a meticulous physical examination, assessing for changes.

5. Selecting adjunctive diagnostic maneuvers as needed, performed with a minimal loss of time.

Bibliography

1. Alyono D, Perry JF: Value of Quantitative Cell Count and Amylase Activity of Peritoneal Lavage Fluid. **Journal of Trauma** 1981;21:345-348.

2. Burke JF: The Effective Period of Preventive Antibiotics in Penetrating Wounds of the Abdomen. **Surgery** 1961;50:161-168.

3. Carroll PR, McAninch JW: Operative Indications in Penetrating Renal Trauma. **Journal of Trauma** 1985;25:587-593.

4. Cass AS: Urethral Injury in the Multiply-injured Patient. **Journal of Trauma** 1984;24:901-906.

5. Committee on Trauma, American College of Surgeons: **Early Care of the Injured Patient.** Philadelphia, WB Saunders Co., 1982, pp 142-182.

6. Dinerman N, Marlin RC: Physician-paramedic Communication, in Moore, Eiseman, and Van Way (Eds.): **Critical Decisions in Trauma**. St. Louis, C.V. Mosby Co, 1984; pp 8-9.

7. Federle MP, Crass RA, Jeffrey B, et al: Computed Tomography in Blunt Abdominal Trauma. **Archives of Surgery** 1982; 117:645-650.

8. Feliciano DV, Bitondo CG, Steed G, et al: Five Hundred Open Taps or Lavages in Patients with Abdominal Stab Wounds. **American Journal of Surgery** 1984;148:772-777.

9. Fischer RP, Beverlin BC, Engrav LH, et al: Diagnostic Peritoneal Lavage: Fourteen Years and 2,586 Patients Later. **American Journal of Surgery** 1978;136:701-704.

10. Flint LM, Brown A, Richardson JD, et al: Definitive Control of Bleeding from Severe Pelvic Fractures. **Annals of Surgery** 1979;189:709-717.

11. Flint LM, McCoy M, Richardson JD and Polk HC Jr: Duodenal Injury-analysis of Common Misconceptions in Diagnosis and Treatment. **Annals of Surgery** 1980;191:697-702.

12. Foley RW, Harris LS, Pilcher DB: Abdominal Injuries in Automobile Accidents: Review of Care of Fatally Injured Patients. **Journal of Trauma** 1977;17:611-615.

13. Fullen WD, Selle JG, Whitely DH, Martin LW, et al: Intramural Duodenal Hematoma. **Annals of Surgery** 1974; 179:549- 556.

14. Gilliland MG, Ward RE, Flynn TC, et al: Peritoneal Lavage and Angiography in Management of Patients with Pelvic Fracture. **American Journal of Surgery** 1982;144:744-747.

15. Griffen WO, Belin RP, Ernst CB, et al: Intravenous Pyelography in Abdominal Trauma. **Journal of Trauma** 1978; 18:387- 392.

16. Hill AC, Schececter, WP, Trunkey DD: Abdominal Trauma and Indications for Exploratory Laparotomy, in Mattox, Moore, and Feliciano (Eds).**Trauma**, Rockville, Appleton-Century-Crofts, 1987.

17. Marx JA, Moore EE, Jorden RC, et al: Limitations of Computed Tomography in the Evaluation of Acute Abdominal Trauma - A Prospective Randomized Comparison with Diagnostic Peritoneal Lavage. **Journal of Trauma** 1985;25:933-937.

18. Kashuk JL, Moore EE, Millikan JS, et al: Major Abdominal Vascular Trauma: A Unified Approach. **Journal of Trauma** 1982;22:672-679.

19. Marx JA, Moore EE, Bar-Or D: Peritoneal Lavage in Small Bowel and Colon Injury: The Value of Enzyme Determinations. **Annals of Emergency Medicine** 1983;12:68-70.

20. Mattox KL, Allen MK, Feliciano DV: Laparotomy in the Emergency Department. **Journal of the American College of Emergency Physicians** 1979;8:180-183.

21. McAlvanah MJ, Shaftan GW: Selective Conservatism in Penetrating Abdominal Wounds: A Continuing Reappraisal. **Journal of Trauma** 1978;18:206-212.

22. Moore EE, Moore JB, Van Duzer-Moore S, et al: Mandatory Laparotomy for Gunshot Wounds Penetrating the Abdomen. **American Journal of Surgery** 1980;140:847-851.

23. Moore EE: Resuscitation and Evaluation of the Injured Patient, in Zuidema, Rutherford, and Ballinger (Eds). **The Management of Trauma.** WB Saunders Co., 1985, pp 1-26.

24. Moore JB, Moore EE, Markovchick VD, et al: Diagnostic Peritoneal Lavage for Abdominal Trauma: Superiority of the Open Technique at the Infraumbilical Ring. **Journal of Trauma** 1981;21:570-572.

25. Moore JB, Moore EE, Thompson JS: Abdominal Injuries Associated with Penetrating Trauma in the Lower Chest. **American Journal of Surgery** 1981;140:724-730.

26. Moreno C, Moore EE, Rosenberger A, et al: Hemorrhage Associated with Major Pelvic Fracture-A Multispecialty Challenge. **Journal of Trauma** 1986. In Press.

27. Mucha P, Farnell MB: Analysis of Pelvic Fracture Management. **Journal of Trauma** 1984;24:379-384.

28. Olsen WR: The Serum Amylase in Blunt Abdominal Trauma. **Journal of Trauma** 1973;13:200-204.

29. Peck JJ, Berne TV: Posterior Abdominal Stab Wounds. **Journal of Trauma** 1981;21:298-306.

30. Pitts RC, Peterson NE: Penetrating Injuries of the Ureter. **Journal of Trauma** 1981;21:978-982.

31. Root HD, Hauser CW, McKinley CR et al: Diagnostic Peritoneal Lavage. **Surgery** 1965;57:633-637.

32. Rothenberger D, Velasco R, Strate R, et al: Open Pelvic Fracture. A Lethal Injury. **Journal of Trauma** 1978;18:184-187.

33. Rothenberg S, Moore EE, Marx, J et al: Selective Management of Blunt Abdominal Trauma in Children—The Triage Role of Peritoneal Lavage. **Journal of Trauma** 1987;27:1101-1106.

34. Takahaski M, Maemura K, Sawada Y, et al: Hyperamylasemia in Critically Injured Patients. **Journal of Trauma** 1980; 20:951-955.

35. Thal ER: Evolution of Peritoneal Lavage and Local Exploration in Lower Chest and Abdominal Stab Wounds. **Journal of Trauma** 1977;17:642-648.

36. Thompson JS, Moore EE, Van Duzer-Moore S, et al: The Evolution of Abdominal Stab Wound Management. **Journal of Trauma** 1980;20:478-484.

37. Trunkey D, Hays RJ, Shires GT: Management of Rectal Trauma. **Journal of Trauma** 1973;13:411-415.

**Chapter 5:
Abdominal
Trauma**

Skill Station VIII: Diagnostic Peritoneal Lavage

This surgical procedure, if performed on a live, anesthetized animal, must be conducted in a USDA Registered Animal Laboratory facility. (See *ATLS Instructor Manual*, Section II, Chapter 10—Animal Laboratory Guidelines and Protocols.)

Equipment

1. Live, anesthetized animals
2. Licensed veterinarian (see guidelines referenced above)
3. Animal trough, ropes (sandbags optional)
4. Animal intubation equipment
   a. Endotracheal tubes
   b. Laryngoscope blade and handle
   c. Respirator with 15-mm adapter
5. Electric shears with #40 blade
6. Tables or instrument stands
7. Needles/syringes
   a. 6-ml syringes with #21- or #25-gauge needles
   b. 12-ml syringes
8. Peritoneal dialysis catheter set-ups
9. Surgical instruments
   a. Disposable scalpels with #10 and #11 blades
   b. Tissue forceps
   c. Allis clamps
   d. Hemostats
10. Antiseptic swabs
11. 500-ml or 1000-ml Ringer's lactate/normal saline with macrodrip and extension tubing
12. Lidocaine with epinephrine
13. Surgical drapes (optional)
14. Surgical garb (gloves, shoe covers, and scrub suits or cover gowns)

**Chapter V:
Abdominal
Trauma**

**Skill
Station
VIII**

1. Upon completion of this station, the participant will be able to discuss the indications and contraindications of peritoneal lavage.

2. Upon completion of this station, the participant will be able to describe the procedure for peritoneal lavage.

3. Performance at this station will allow the participant to practice and demonstrate the technique of peritoneal lavage.

4. Upon completion of this station, the participant will be able to discuss complications of this procedure.

The skill procedure for peritoneal lavage is performed via the open-technique method to avoid injury to underlying structures as may occur with the use of the trocar technique.

Objectives

Chapter 5:
Abdominal
Trauma

Skill
Station
VIII

Skill Procedure

Diagnostic Peritoneal Lavage

I. Peritoneal Lavage Technique

A. Decompress the urinary bladder by inserting a urinary catheter.

B. Decompress the stomach by inserting a nasogastric tube.

C. Surgically prep the abdomen (eg, costal margin to the pubic area and flank to flank, anteriorly).

D. Inject local anesthetic midline and one-third the distance from the umbilicus to the symphysis pubis. Use lidocaine with epinephrine to avoid blood contamination from skin and subcutaneous tissue.

E. Vertically incise the skin and subcutaneous tissues to the fascia.

F. Incise the fascia and peritoneum, and grasp the fascial edges with clamps to provide countertraction.

G. Insert a peritoneal dialysis catheter into the peritoneal cavity.

H. After inserting the catheter into the peritoneum, advance the catheter into the pelvis.

I. Connect the dialysis catheter to a syringe and aspirate.

J. If gross blood is not obtained, instill 10 ml/kg (body weight) of warmed Ringer's lactate/normal saline (up to 1 liter) into the peritoneum through the intravenous tubing attached to the dialysis catheter.

K. Gentle agitation of the abdomen distributes the fluid throughout the peritoneal cavity and increases mixing with the blood.

L. If the patient is stable, allow the fluid to remain 5 to 10 minutes before siphoning off. This is done by putting the Ringer's lactate/normal saline container on the floor and allowing the peritoneal fluid to drain from the ab-domen (this may take 20 to 30 minutes). Make sure the container is vented to promote flow of the fluid from the abdomen.

M. After the fluid has returned, send a sample to the lab for erythrocyte and leukocyte counts (unspun). 100,000 erythrocytes per cubic millimeter or more and greater that 500 leukocytes per cubic millimeter indicate a positive test and the need for surgical intervention.

N. Negative lavage indicates the absence of significant free blood in the peritoneal cavity. However, it **does not** rule out retroperitoneal injuries, ie, pancreas or duodenum, isolated hollow visceral perforation, or diaphragmatic tears.

Chapter V:
Abdominal
Trauma

Skill
Station
VIII

Complications of Peritoneal Lavage

1. Hemorrhage, secondary to injection of local anesthetic, incision of the skin, or subcutaneous tissues providing a false-positive study.

2. Peritonitis due to intestinal perforation from the catheter.

3. Laceration of urinary bladder (if bladder not evacuated prior to procedure).

5. Injury to other abdominal and retroperitoneal structures requiring operative care.

6. Wound infection at the lavage site (late complication).

Chapter 6:
Head Trauma

Objectives:

Upon completion of this topic, the physician will be able to demonstrate the techniques of assessment and explain the emergency management of head trauma.

Specifically, the physician will be able to:

A. Review specific principles of anatomy and physiology related to head injuries.

B. Identify and discuss the principles of general management of the unconscious, traumatized patient, and delayed complications.

C. Outline the method of evaluating head injuries using a minineurological examination.

D. Identify and discuss management techniques for specific types of head injuries.

E. Demonstrate the ability to assess various types of head, maxillofacial, and neck injuries, using a head-trauma manikin.

F. Discuss clinical signs and outline priorities for the initial management of injuries identified in the assessment.

**Chapter 6:
Head
Trauma**

American College of Surgeons

I. Introduction

Because a head injury occurs every 15 seconds, and a patient dies of a head injury every 12 minutes, a physician dealing with trauma is confronted with a head injury patient almost every day. Approximately 50% of all trauma deaths are associated with head injury, and more than 60% of vehicular trauma deaths are due to head injury. Because of the immense importance of head injury, the physician who sees patients soon after injury, but is not expert in the comprehensive management of head injuries, must develop a practical knowledge of the initial care of these patients. A neurosurgeon may not be immediately available when a patient with a central nervous system injury is first seen. One of the most important responsibilities of physicians initially evaluating such a patient is therefore in the management of ventilation and hypovolemia, thereby obviating potential secondary brain damage. A system that incorporates consultation with a neurosurgeon, whose opinion may modify the management of such a patient, is therefore essential. Early transfer of appropriate cases will substantially reduce morbidity and mortality.

When conferring with a neurosurgical consultant about a patient with a head injury, the physician should relay the following patient information:

1. Age of patient and mechanism of injury.

2. Respiratory and cardiovascular status.

3. Results of the neurological examination, especially the level of consciousness, the pupillary reactions, and the presence of lateralized extremity weakness.

4. Presence and type of noncerebral injuries.

5. The results of diagnostic studies, if obtained.

Obtaining diagnostic studies, ie, a computed tomography (CT) scan or skull roentgenograms, should not delay treatment, neurosurgical consultation, or patient transfer.

II. Anatomy and Physiology

As with all other aspects of medicine, the basis for a rational decision is the integration of the knowledge of anatomy and physiology with the history and physical examination. A short review of these subjects follows.

A. Scalp

The scalp is made up of five layers of tissue covering the bone of the top of the skull (calvarium): 1) skin, 2) subcutaneous tissue, 3) galea aponeurotica, 4) a layer of loose areolar tissue, and 5) periosteum, the "pericranium." The loose areolar tissue, separating the galea from the pericranium, is subject to the commonly encountered subgaleal hematomas, large flaps caused by injury and "scalping" injuries. Because of the scalp's generous blood supply, bleeding from a scalp laceration can result in major blood loss, especially in children.

B. Skull

The skull is composed of the cranial vault (calvarium) and the base. The calvarium is especially thin in the temporal regions. The base of the skull is irregular and rough, allowing injury to occur as the brain moves within the skull during acceleration and deceleration.

C. Meninges

The **dura** is a tough, fibrous membrane that adheres firmly to the internal surface of the skull. Because it is not attached to the underlying arachnoid, a potential space (the **subdural space**) exists into which hemorrhage can occur–usually from veins that traverse the space (bridging veins). In certain places the dura splits into two surfaces forming venous sinuses that provide the major venous drainage from the brain. The midline (superior) sagittal sinus is especially vulnerable to injury.

Meningeal arteries lie between the dura and the internal surface of the skull (**epidural space**). The courses of these arteries may be visible on plain skull roentgenograms, if the vessels groove the inner surface of the skull. Laceration of these arteries may result in an epidural hematoma.

Beneath the dura is a second meningeal layer, the thin transparent **arachnoid**. The third layer, the **pia**, is firmly attached to the brain cortex. Between the arachnoid and the pia (**subarachnoid space**), the cerebrospinal fluid circulates. Hemorrhage into this space is, by definition, subarachnoid hemorrhage.

D. Brain

The brain consists of the cerebrum, the cerebellum, and the brainstem. The **cerebrum** is composed of right and left hemispheres that are separated by the falx, a dural reflection. The left hemisphere usually contains the language centers and is often referred to as the dominant hemisphere. The **frontal lobe** is concerned with emotions and motor function, the **occipital lobe** with vision, and the **parietal lobe** with sensory function. The **temporal lobe** regulates certain memory functions but can be a relatively silent region on the right side.

The brain can be compared to a funnel. The two cerebral hemispheres comprise the funnel portion. The brain stem, the major neural pathways to and from the hemispheres, comprises the neck of the funnel. The **brain stem** is composed of the midbrain, the pons, and the medulla. The midbrain and upper pons contain the **reticular activating system**, which is responsible for an "awake" state. Vital cardiorespiratory centers reside in the lower brain stem, the **medulla**, which then continues to form the spinal cord. The **cerebellum,** which controls movement, coordination, and balance, surrounds the pons and medulla in the posterior fossa.

E. Cerebrospinal Fluid

Cerebrospinal fluid is produced by the choroid plexus and is discharged into the ventricles of the brain. The fluid leaves the ventricular cavities to circulate through the subarachnoid space.

F. Tentorium

The tentorium divides the head into the supratentorial compartment (comprising the anterior and middle fossae of the skull) and the infratentorial compartment (containing the posterior fossa). The midbrain courses from the cerebrum through the large aperture (incisura) in the tentorium. The third cranial nerve also passes along this opening. Any pathological process that rapidly increases supratentorial pressure, most commonly hemorrhage or edema, can force the medial aspect of the temporal lobe (the uncus) through this opening. The result (uncal or tentorial herniation) causes compression of the third nerve, producing an ipsilateral and dilated, fixed pupil. Contralateral spastic weakness of the arm and leg, caused by compression of the corticospinal (pyramidal) tract within the cerebral peduncle on the side of herniation, is also an integral component of uncal herniation.

G. Consciousness

Alteration of consciousness is the hallmark of brain injury.

Two types of brain injury–bilateral injury to the cerebral cortices, and injury to the reticular activating system of the brainstem–can produce unconsciousness. Increased intracranial pressure and decreased cerebral blood flow, regardless of the cause, can also depress the level of consciousness.

H. Intracranial Pressure

The final common pathway in many severe injuries is related to increased intracranial pressure. Intracranial pressure problems arise because the size of the various compartments of the brain are fixed by the surrounding rigid skull. Therefore, any increase in volume (as from a hematoma) in one compartment can increase pressure. There is some give to this system, because cerebrospinal fluid (CSF) and blood can be squeezed out of the head. Trouble begins when all possible CSF has been eliminated, and the blood volume has been reduced to as low a level as is compatible with normal brain function.

When all normal compensatory measures are exhausted, further small increases in intracranial volume cause very large increases in intracranial pressure, resulting in diminution of cerebral perfusion pressure. If this situation continues, intracranial pressure rises at the expense of cerebral blood flow and results in brain ischemia. High intracranial pressure can cause alterations in the level of consciousness; coma; hypertension; bradycardia; and ultimately, brain death. Brain death occurs when intracranial pressure approaches systemic arterial pressure, thus preventing any blood flow to the brain.

III. Assessment of Head Injuries

A. History

To make the correct management decisions, it is helpful to know what kind of head injury can result from a certain kind of trauma. The cause is usually obvious, but even though a patient may appear to be in good neurological condition, mechanism-of-injury risk factors should be assessed in deciding how and where to treat the patient (See Chapter 12–Stabilization and Transport). For example, simply knowing that the patient was injured in a fall instead of a vehicular crash quadruples that patient's risk of having an intracranial hematoma.

Prehospital personnel should question observers at the scene about the patient's condition immediately after the incident. Information obtained by ambulance personnel should be documented in writing and provided to the hospital personnel when the patient is delivered to the emergency department. **The importance of initial assessment is emphasized because it provides the baseline for sequential reassessment, which is the critical basis for many subsequent decisions in management of the patient.**

Because many factors influence the neurological evaluation, documentation of the cardiorespiratory status must accompany the neurological examination. **Airway, breathing, and circulatory control and management must take priority.** Care must be exercised in attributing changes in the patient's mental status to head injury if the systolic blood pressure is less than 60 mmHg or systemic hypoxemia exists. Similarly, a drug screen for alcohol and other nervous system depressants must be obtained, so that toxic factors that may influence head injury assessment are taken into account.

B. Assessment of Vital Signs

Although brain injury may alter the vital signs, it is very difficult to be sure that changes in the vital signs are due to head injury and not to other factors. Some useful clinical rules include:

1. **Never presume that brain injury is the cause of hypotension.** Although bleeding from scalp lacerations can cause hemorrhagic shock, intracranial bleeding cannot produce shock, except very rarely in infants. Hypotension arising from brain injury is a terminal event, resulting from failure of medullary centers.

2. The combination of progressive hypertension associated with bradycardia and diminished respiratory rate (Cushing response) is a specific response to an acute and potentially lethal rise in intracranial pressure. In head injury, the course is usually a lesion demanding immediate operative intervention.

3. Hypertension alone or in combination with hyperthermia may reflect central autonomic dysfunction caused by certain types of brain injury.

C. Minineurological Examination

The AVPU mneumonic is supplemented by a minineurological examination that is directed toward determining the presence and severity of gross neurological deficits, especially those that may require urgent operation. The AVPU method, completed in the primary survey, describes the patient's level of consciousness. (See Chapter 1–Initial Assessment and Management.)

The minineurological examination should be conducted repeatedly for any patient with a head injury. The examination assesses: 1) level of consciousness, 2) pupillary function, and 3) lateralized extremity weakness. **Generally,** a patient with abnormalities of all three components will have a mass lesion that may require surgery.

1. Level of consciousness

The Glasgow Coma Scale (GCS) provides a quantitative measure of the patient's level of consciousness. The GCS is the sum of scores for three areas of assessment: 1) eye opening, 2) best motor response, and 3) verbal response. Each is graded separately.

a. Eye-opening response (E score)

Scoring of eye-opening is not valid if the eyes are swollen shut. This fact must be documented.

1) Spontaneous–already open with blinking (normal): **E= four (4) points.**

2) To speech–not necessarily to a request for eye opening: **E= three(3) points.**

3) To pain–stimulus should not be applied to the face: **E= two (2) points.**

4) None: **E = one (1) point.**

b. Best motor response (M score)

The **best** response obtained for any extremity is recorded even though worse responses may be present in other extremities. The worst motor activity is also important but is not used for the GCS; worst response should be noted separately. For patients not following verbal command, a painful stimulus is applied to the fingernail or toenail.

1) Obeys–moves limb to command and pain is not required: **M = six (6) points.**

2) Localizes–changing the location of the pain stimulus causes purposeful motion toward the stimulus: **M = five (5) points.**

3) Withdraws–pulls away from painful stimulus: **M = four (4) points.**

4) Abnormal flexion–decorticate posture: **M = three (3) points.**

5) Extensor response–decerebrate posture: **M = two (2) points.**

6) No movement: **M = one (1) point.**

c. Verbal response (V score)

Scoring of verbal response is invalid if speech is impossible, for example, in the presence of endotracheal intubation. This circumstance must be documented.

1) Oriented–knows name, age, etc: **V = five (5) points.**

2) Confused conversation–still answers questions: **V = four (4) points**.

3) Inappropriate words–speech is either exclamatory or random, but recognizable words are produced: **V = three (3) points**.

4) Incomprehensible sounds–grunts and groans are produced, but no actual words are uttered; do not confuse with partial respiratory obstruction: **V = two (2) points**.

5) None: **V = (1) point.**

The Glasgow Coma Scale itself can be used to categorize patients:

1) Coma

A patient in **coma is defined as having no eye opening (E=1), and no ability to follow commands (M=1 to 5), and no word verbalizations (V=1 to 2).** This means that all patients with a GCS < 8 and most of those with a GCS = 8 are in coma. Patients with a GCS > 8 are not in coma.

2) Head injury severity

On the basis of the GCS, patients are classified as having:

a) Severe head injury if GCS ≤ 8.
b) Moderate head injury if GCS is 9 to 12.
c) Minor head injury if GCS is 13 to 15.

2. Assessment of pupillary function

The pupils are evaluated for their equality and response to bright light. A difference in pupil diameters of more than 1 mm is abnormal. Even though eye injury may be present, intracranial injury must be excluded. Light reactivity must be evaluated for the briskness of response; a more sluggish response may indicate an intracranial injury.

3. Lateralized extremity weakness

Spontaneous movements are observed for equality. If spontaneous motion is minimal, the response to a painful stimulus is assessed. A delay in onset of movement, less movement, or need for more stimulus on one side is significant. Often, the motor component of the Glasgow Coma Scale can be used to score the best and the worst extremity movement. A clearly lateralized weakness suggests an intracranial mass lesion.

4. Purposes of neurological examination

The purposes of the minineurological examination are to determine the severity of the brain injury, and detect any neurological deterioration. The Glasgow Coma Scale can be used to categorize injuries as mild, moderate, and severe. Irrespective of the Glasgow Coma Scale, a patient is considered to have a severe head injury if he exhibits **any** of the following:

a. Unequal pupils

b. Unequal motor examination

c. An open head injury with leaking cerebrospinal fluid or exposed brain tissue.

d. Neurological deterioration

e. Depressed skull fracture

A change in the Glasgow Coma Scale score of two or more points clearly means the patient has deteriorated. A decrease of three or more points is a catastrophic deterioration that demands immediate treatment if the cause is remediable. However, these changes are rather gross and are often preceded by more subtle signs of deterioration. Neurological deterioration of special concern include the following:

f. Increase in severity of a headache or an extraordinarily severe headache

g. An increase in the size of one pupil

h. Development of weakness on one side

It cannot be overemphasized that the initial neurologic examination is only the beginning. The initial findings are only the reference with which to compare results of repeated neurologic examinations to determine whether a patient is deteriorating or improving. **All previous efforts will go to waste if signs of neurologic deterioration are not appreciated.** The brain cannot withstand unrelieved compression for very long before brain damage is irretrievable . The neurological assessment is designed to detect this secondary brain damage so timely treatment can be initiated.

D. Special Assessment

1. Skull roentgenograms

Skull roentgenograms are of little value in the early management of patients with obvious head injuries, except in cases of penetrating injuries. The unconscious patient should have skull roentgenograms **only** if precise care of the cardiorespiratory system and continuing reassessment can be assured. Physical examination is usually more valuable than skull roentgenograms. For example, when there is a scalp laceration, a skull fracture can often be diagnosed by visual inspection and/or careful palpation with a gloved finger. Clinical signs of basal fractures are more useful than radiographs of the skull base in diagnosing fracture. For a patient with a minor head injury, skull roentgenograms may be recommended before considering the discharge of a patient from the emergency department.

2. Computerized tomography

The computed tomography (CT) scan has revolutionized diagnosis in patients with head injuries and is the diagnostic procedure of choice for patients who have or are suspected of having a serious head injury. Although not perfect, the CT scan is capable of showing the exact location and size of most mass lesions. Specific diagnosis allows more precise planning of definitive care, including operation. The CT scan has supplanted less specific and more invasive tests such as cerebral angiography.

Except for patients with trivial head injuries, **all head-injured patients will require CT scanning** at some time. The more serious the injury, the earlier and more emergent is the need for the scan. Consequently, injured patients seen first at facilities without computed tomography capability may require transfer to more sophisticated hospitals.

Once initial resuscitation has been undertaken and the need for a CT scan determined, care must be taken to: 1) maintain adequate resuscitation during the scan, and 2) assure the best possible quality of the scan. The patient must be attended constantly in the CT suite to closely monitor his vital signs, and initiate immediate treatment should the patient's status deteriorate.

Patient movement results in artifacts and a poor-quality scan. This artifact may mask significant intracranial lesions requiring urgent surgical intervention. Movement artifact can be eliminated by sedating restless or uncooperative patients. However, extreme caution must be exercised to avoid sedating patients whose restlessness or "lack of cooperation" is a clinical manifestation of hypoxia. Often endotracheal intubation with controlled ventilation becomes necessary if the scan is considered mandatory, and the patient can be rendered motionless only with paralyzing drugs.

3. Other tests

Lumbar puncture, electroencephalogram, and isotope scanning have no role in the acute management of head trauma.

Certain reflexes can reflect the integrity of a portion of the brain stem neural pathways. Although these may permit more specific diagnosis in some instances, their use can be hazardous, their interpretation difficult; and they add little to the emergency management of the patient. They are best left to the neurosurgical consultant.

IV. Specific Types of Head Injury

After initial assessment and resuscitation, the emergency management of the patient with a head injury is aimed at: 1) establishing a specific anatomic diagnosis of the head injury, 2) assuring the metabolic needs of the brain, and 3) preventing secondary brain damage from treatable causes of elevated intracranial pressure. The need to prevent systemic causes of secondary brain injury, notably hypoxia, ischemia, and hyperthermia, is axiomatic.

Head injuries include: 1) skull fractures, 2) diffuse brain injuries, and 3) focal injuries. The pathophysiology, severity, need for urgent treatment, and outcome are different in each group. A review of these head injuries aids in making and simplifing the initial diagnosis.

A. Skull Fractures

Skull fractures are common, but do not, by themselves, cause neurologic disability. Many severe brain injuries occur without skull fracture, and many skull fractures are not associated with severe brain injury. Although identifying a skull fracture is important, diagnosing a brain injury does not depend on it. Searching for a skull fracture should never delay patient management. Attention should be directed to the brain injury. The significance of a skull fracture is that it identifies the patient with a higher probability of having or developing an intracranial hematoma. For this reason, all patients with skull fractures should be admitted for observation. All patients with skull fractures require neurosurgical consultation.

1. Linear, nondepressed fractures

Linear skull fractures are often seen on the roentgenogram as a lucent line. They may also be stellate. Linear skull fractures require no specific treatment, and management is directed toward the underlying brain injury. Fractures across vascular arterial grooves or suture lines should raise suspicion of the possibility of epidural hemorrhage.

2. Depressed skull fractures

Depressed skull fractures may or may not be neurosurgical emergencies. Management is directed toward the underlying brain injury. To reduce the risk of possible sequelae, such as a seizure disorder, any fragment depressed more than the thickness of the skull may require operative elevation of the bony fragment.

3. Open skull fractures

By definition, open skull fractures have a direct communication between a scalp laceration and the cerebral substance, because the dura is torn. This condition can be diagnosed if brain is visible or if cerebrospinal fluid (CSF) is leaking from the wound. Open fractures require early operative intervention, with elevation or removal of the fragments and closure of the dura. Compound fractures differ, because the dural membrane protecting the brain is intact. These fractures may require early operative intervention with elevation or removal of the fragments and exploration for tears of the dura.

4. Basal skull fractures

These fractures are often not apparent on skull films. Indirectly, intracranial air or an opaque sphenoid sinus give clues.

The diagnosis is based on physical findings such as cerebrospinal fluid leaking from the ear (otorrhea) or the nose (rhinorrhea). When cerebrospinal fluid is mixed with blood, it may be difficult to detect. An aid is the "ring sign", detected by allowing a drop of the fluid to fall onto a piece of filter paper. If cerebrospinal fluid is present, blood remains in the center, and one or more concentric rings of clearer fluid develop.

Ecchymosis in the mastoid region (Battle's sign) also indicates a basal skull fracture, as does blood behind the tympanic membrane (hemotympanum). Cribriform plate fractures are often associated with periorbital ecchymosis (raccoon eyes). These signs may take several hours to appear, and may be absent immediately after injury. Whenever a frontal basal skull fracture is present, danger exists of inadvertent intracranial intubation with the insertion of a nasogastric tube. If this catastrophe occurs, the patient usually dies.

B. Diffuse Brain Injuries

Diffuse brain injuries are produced when rapid head motions (acceleration or deceleration) cause widespread interruption of brain function in most areas of the brain. Often, as with concussion, the disturbance of neural function is temporary. But with more severe injuries (diffuse axonal injury), microscopic structural damage throughout the brain may cause permanent problems. It is important to try to distinguish these injuries from focal injuries, because diffuse brain injuries do not have mass lesions requiring emergency surgery.

1. Concussion

Concussion is a brain injury accompanied by brief loss of neurologic function. In its more mild forms, it may cause only temporary confusion or amnesia. More commonly, concussion causes temporary loss of consciousness. The period of unconsciousness is usually short, but more severe forms exist. Many neurologic abnormalities may be described in the first few minutes after concussion, but these disappear quickly, usually before the patient gets to a medical facility. **Therefore, any neurologic abnormality observed in the patient should not be attributed to a concussion.**

Most patients with a concussion will be awake or awakening when seen in the emergency department, even though some mental confusion may persist. After the confusion clears, the patient may be capable of describing portions of his accident, but does not remember the actual impact. The patient may complain of headache, dizziness, or nausea, but the mini-neurologic examination will not show localizing signs. These patients should be observed in the hospital and then at home only if their mental state clears completely. Patients sustaining a severe concussion should be admitted for observation, because of the potential for associated serious brain injuries. The decision to admit the patient should be based on the length of unconsciousness and the reliability of the individuals with whom the patient resides. A rule of thumb is that if a patient has been unconscious for five to fifteen minutes or more, he should be observed in the hospital for 24 hours. The duration of amnesia and/or retrograde amnesia also must be considered. If the patient is under the age of 12, it is best to admit for observation. Persistent vomiting and/or convulsions may occur. Any patient whose confusion does not clear completely **must** be admitted.

2. Diffuse axonal injury

Diffuse axonal injury (DAI)–often called brain stem injury, closed head injury, or diffuse injury–is similar to severe concussion, and is characterized by prolonged coma, often lasting days to weeks. DAI is a frequent injury, occurring in 44% of coma-producing head injuries.

Overall mortality is 33%. In its most severe form, DAI has a 50% mortality. Diffuse axonal injury results primarily in microscopic damage that is scattered widely throughout the brain, and therefore does not require surgery. Although the length of coma cannot be determined in the emergency department, recognition of DAI is important because it may mimic other injuries that do require emergency surgery. The diagnosis is justified when an emergency CT scan shows no mass lesion in a patient who remains deeply comatose, often with decerebrate or decorticate posturing. Autonomic dysfunction producing high fever, hypertension, and sweating is common. The patient should be transferred to a facility equipped to care for long-term coma patients.

C. Focal Injuries

Focal injuries are those in which macroscopic damage occurs in a relatively local area. They consist of contusions, hemorrhages, and hematomas. These injuries may require emergency surgery because of their mass effects. **Diagnostic efforts during the early postinjury period are primarily aimed at diagnosing focal lesions, because they are treatable and frequently require emergency operative intervention.**

1. Contusion

Cerebral contusions can be single or multiple, small or large, and the patient may therefore present in several ways. Most commonly, contusions are associated with serious concussions characterized by longer periods of coma and mental confusion or obtundation. Contusions can occur beneath an area of impact (coup contusions) or in areas remote from impact (contrecoup contusions). The tips of the frontal and temporal lobes are especially common sites of contusion. The contusion itself may produce focal neurologic deficit if it occurs near the sensory or motor areas of the brain, but a deficit may not be apparent if the contusion is elsewhere. If the contusion is large or associated with pericontusional edema, the mass effect may cause herniation and brain stem compression, resulting in secondary or delayed neurological deterioration.

Before the era of computed tomography, contusions were diagnosed clinically for patients who were unconscious for long periods. Predictably, this practice resulted in many incorrect diagnoses. Today, a CT scan of the head will determine with certainty the presence, location, and size of contusions.

Patients sustaining cerebral contusion should be admitted to the hospital for observation, because delayed edema or swelling around the contusion may cause neurologic deterioration. Contusions require surgery only if they cause substantial mass effect, but careful observation is necessary to detect patients with delayed bleeding into the contusion. This factor is especially important for patients with measurable blood ethanol levels, because acutely or chronically alcoholic patients have a high incidence of delayed bleeding into their contusions.

2. Intracranial hemorrhages

Intracranial hemorrhages can be classified as meningeal or brain hemorrhages. Due to great variation in location, size, and rapidity of bleeding, there is no typical picture. Computed tomography has made the diagnosis and localization very precise. It must be stressed that epidural hematoma and temporal lobe intracerebral hematoma can mimic each other, because the symptoms and the clinical findings are usually that of tentorial herniation, characteristically seen in epidural hemorrhage.

a. Meningeal hemorrhage

1) Acute epidural hemorrhage

Epidural bleeding almost always occurs from a tear in a dural artery, usually the middle meningeal artery. A small percentage may occur from a tear in the dural sinus. Although epidural hemorrhage is relatively rare (0.5% in unselected head injuries and 0.9% of coma-producing head injuries), it must be considered because it may be rapidly fatal. Such arterial tears are usually associated with linear skull fractures over the parietal or temporal areas that cross the grooves of the middle meningeal artery; however, **this injury is not an absolute requirement for the diagnosis.**

The signs and symptoms of a typical epidural hemorrhage are: 1) loss of consciousness (concussion) followed by an intervening lucid interval (the lucid period may not be a return to full consciousness), 2) a secondary depression of consciousness, and 3) the development of hemiparesis on the opposite side. A dilated and fixed pupil on the same side as the impact area is a hallmark of this injury. (Less frequently, the dilated, fixed pupil may be on the side opposite the hematoma, or the hemiparesis may be on the same side as the hematoma.) While the patient is lucid, he may not be entirely symptom-free, usually complains of a severe localized headache, and is sleepy.

This injury requires immediate surgical intervention. If treated early, prognosis is usually excellent, because the underlying brain injury is often not serious. Outcome is directly related to the status of the patient before surgery. For patients not in coma, the mortality from epidural hematoma approximates zero. For those in light coma it is 9%, and for patients in deep coma it is 20%. Secondary brain injury will occur rapidly if the hematoma is not quickly evacuated.

2) Acute subdural hematoma

Subdural hematomas are also life-threatening and are much more common than epidural hematomas (30% of severe head injuries). They most commonly occur from rupture of bridging veins between the cerebral cortex and dura, but also can be seen with lacerations of the brain or cortical arteries. A skull fracture may or may not be present. In addition to the problems caused by the mass of the subdural blood, underlying primary brain injury is often severe. The prognosis is often dismal, and the mortality remains 60%. However, recent studies demonstrate improved outcome if the hematoma is evacuated very early.

3) Subarachnoid hemorrhage

This type of hemorrhage results in bloody CSF and meningeal irritation. The patient usually complains of a headache and/or photophobia. No immediate treatment is needed, and the hemorrhage alone is not life-threatening. A lumbar puncture is not needed, because the diagnosis can be made with a CT scan.

b. Brain hemorrhages and lacerations

1) Intracerebral hematomas

Hemorrhages within the brain substance can occur in any location. Computed tomography provides a more precise diagnosis. Many small, deep intracerebral hemorrhages are associated with other brain injuries (especially DAI). The neurological deficits depend upon these associated injuries and the region(s) involved, the size of the hemorrhage, and whether or not bleeding continues. Hemiplegia may occur. Occipital hemorrhages can cause visual defects. Intraventricular and intracerebellar hemorrhages are associated with a high mortality rate.

2) Impalement injuries

All foreign bodies protruding from the skull should be left in place until they can be removed by a neurosurgeon as a formal operation. Roentgenograms of the skull are required to determine the object's angle and depth of penetration.

3) Bullet wounds

The larger the caliber and the higher the velocity of the bullet, the more likely death will occur. Through-and-through and side-to-side injuries, and those lower in the brain, tend to be ominous. The outcome is related to the patient's condition. Patients in coma have a very high mortality. Skull films and a CT scan help plan the surgical approach when operation is deemed necessary. Entrance and exit wounds should be covered with antiseptic-soaked dressings until definitive neurosurgical care is provided. A bullet that does not penetrate the skull may still result in intracranial injury, and such patients require a CT scan.

V. Emergency Management of Head Injuries

A. Establishing a Specific Diagnosis

The immediate purpose of a specific diagnosis is to determine which patients need an emergency or urgent neurosurgical operation. **This is an issue that demands early participation by the neurosurgical consultant.** The patients requiring emergency surgery are those with massive depressed or open skull fractures and those with large focal mass lesions. The former category is usually obvious, but the latter must be distinguished from diffuse brain injuries where no mass lesion exists.

1. Rules of thumb in assessing the need for surgery

Injuries requiring surgery are likely to occur in different circumstances than injuries not requiring surgery. Therefore, a gross estimate of a patient's potential need for surgery can be based on knowledge concerning three factors: 1) whether the patient is comatose, 2) whether the trauma was vehicular or nonvehicular, and 3) whether there is a lateralized motor deficit. (See Table 1.)

Thus, irrespective of the patient's clinical status, head injuries resulting from nonvehicular accidents are much more likely to require emergency surgery than vehicle occupants or pedestrians. Victims of falls and assaults develop focal mass lesions more frequently; vehicular injuries tend to produce greater numbers of diffuse brain injuries that do not require surgery. If all one knows is that the patient is comatose, has unequal movements, and was not an occupant in the vehicle or a pedestrian, the odds are at least four to one that he needs surgery. Although these guidelines cannot govern management of specific patients, they are extremely useful to remember.

Table 1
Approximate Percent of Patients Who May Require Surgery
(Excludes patients with minor injury who are neurologically normal.)

| | Not in Coma | | | Comatose | |
	Motor Equal	Unequal	Motor	Equal	Unequal
Vehicular	20%	40%		20%	30%
Nonvehicular	40%	70%		60%	80%

2. Diagnostic triage system

Based on the minineurological examination, practical and a systematic approach can be established for diagnosing patients with head injuries. It must be understood that this scheme is only a guideline (see Figure 1). Because of the complexity and multiplicity of brain injuries, this system is not and cannot be either foolproof or all-inclusive. However, this system offers one approach to determining not only the initial diagnosis, but also the severity of injury, so that emergency treatment decisions can be made.

The first priority is determining the level of consciousness, based on the Glasgow Coma Scale. If a patient has a score equal to or less than eight, the physician must immediately determine: 1) whether the pupils are unequal, or 2) whether there is a lateralized motor deficit. If either of these exist, **a large focal lesion (epidural, subdural, or intracerebral hematoma, or large contusion) must be presumed present.** Preparation must be made for emergency operation to evacuate the lesion. Simultaneously, efforts must be taken to decrease the intracranial pressure. Presumptive evidence of a progressive lesion capable of producing

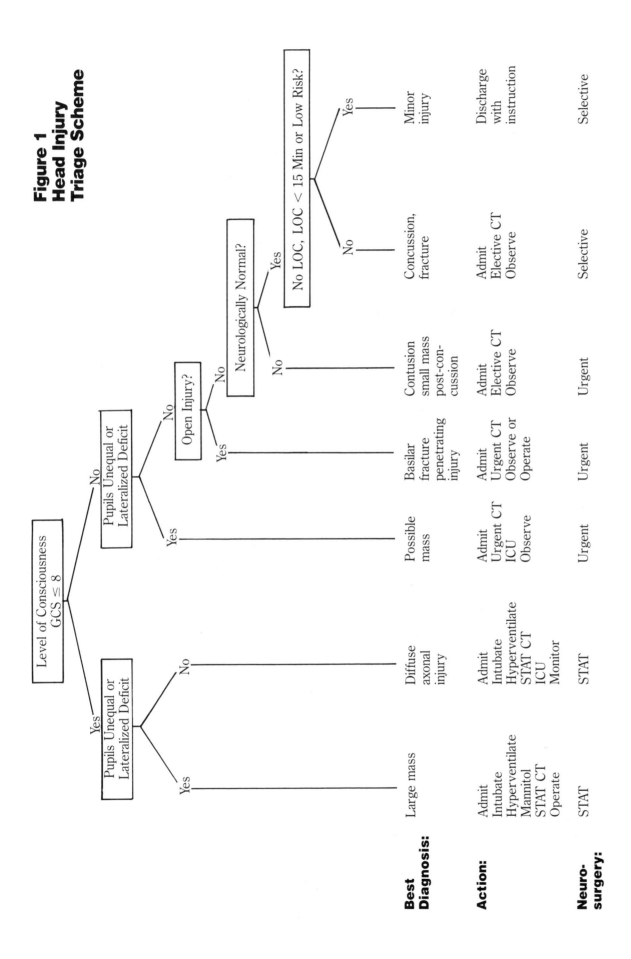

**Figure 1
Head Injury
Triage Scheme**

	Large mass	Diffuse axonal injury	Possible mass	Basilar fracture penetrating injury	Contusion small mass post-concussion	Concussion, fracture	Minor injury
Best Diagnosis:	Large mass	Diffuse axonal injury	Possible mass	Basilar fracture penetrating injury	Contusion small mass post-concussion	Concussion, fracture	Minor injury
Action:	Admit Intubate Hyperventilate Mannitol STAT CT Operate	Admit Intubate Hyperventilate STAT CT ICU Monitor	Admit Urgent CT ICU Observe	Admit Urgent CT Observe or Operate	Admit Elective CT Observe	Admit Elective CT Observe	Discharge with instruction
Neuro-surgery:	STAT	STAT	Urgent	Urgent	Urgent	Selective	Selective

lethal brain herniation (usually an epidural hematoma) is one of the few neurosurgical emergencies in the injured that may require operative intervention within minutes.

A comatose patient with equal pupils and motor responses may still have a surgical mass lesion but is more likely to have diffuse axonal injury, acute brain swelling, or cerebral ischemia. After immediate measures have been taken to reduce intracranial pressure, an emergency CT is needed to exclude a mass lesion.

A patient who is not comatose (ie, GCS > 8) still may harbor an injury requiring operation. If pupillary asymmetry or lateralized weakness is present, the patient must be suspected to have a focal lesion that is not (yet) of sufficient size to compress the brain stem and cause coma. A CT scan is urgently required. If the pupils and movements are equal, the presence or absence of an open head injury must be determined by a search for CSF leaking from the nose, ears, or a scalp wound.

If there is no open injury (in the noncomatose patient who has equal pupils and movements), a complete neurological examination must be performed. If the examination is not normal, a focal lesion must be excluded by CT scan. If the examination is normal, and the patient has been unconscious only briefly and is in the low-risk group for an intracranial lesion (see Table 2), discharge may be considered after appropriate instructions are given to patient. If any of these conditions are not met, the patient should be admitted for postconcussion observation. **Remember, a normal neurological examination includes a normal mental status examination.** No patient with signs of head injury should be discharged because he is intact except for being intoxicated. **Do not presume that altered mental status is due to alcohol.** The patient should be observed until his mental status is completely normal, or he should be admitted for observation.

B. Emergency Management

Once a working diagnosis is established, treatment must be commenced; urgency of treatment depends on the nature and severity of injury. Emergency treatment of the seriously injured patient is aimed at protecting the brain from further (secondary) insults by: 1) maintaining adequate cerebral metabolism, and 2) preventing and treating intracranial hypertension.

1. Maintenance of cerebral metabolic needs

Cerebral ischemia or hypoxia result in insufficient substrate delivery to the injured brain. These conditions are present in over 90% of patients who die from head trauma, are associated with poor outcome, and are the most important preventable complications of head injury.

The principal metabolic requirements of the brain are oxygen and glucose, which are normally used at extremely high rates. The injured brain usually has a lowered cerebral metabolism and therefore requires less oxygen and glucose. However, the damaged brain is more susceptible to the lack of these substrates, and thus temporary severe or prolonged moderate deprivation causes worse damage than in the uninjured brain.

Therefore, emergency management of head injury includes maintenance of adequate cerebral metabolic fuels.

Table 2
Relative Risk of Intracranial Lesion

Low Risk Group	Moderate Risk	High Risk
Asymptomatic	Change of consciousness	Depressed consciousness
Headache	Progressive headache	Focal signs
Dizziness	Alcohol or drug intoxication	Decreasing consciousness
Scalp hematoma	Unreliable history	Penetrating injury
Scalp laceration	Age > 2 years	Palpable, depressed fracture
Scalp contusion	Posttraumatic seizure	
Scalp abrasion	Vomiting	
Absence of moderate or high-risk criteria	Posttraumatic amnesia	
	Multiple trauma	
	Serious facial injury	
	Signs of basilar fracture	
	Possible skull penetration	
	Possible depressed fracture	
	Suspected child abuse	

The physician must assure delivery of adequate levels of glucose and oxygen to the brain. Delivery of these substrates depends on their arterial concentrations and the blood flow to the brain. Blood glucose concentration is not a common problem in trauma, but if it is, correction with supplemental intravenous glucose is needed.

Oxygen content depends on arterial hemoglobin and oxygen concentrations. Arterial oxygen concentration can be assessed with blood gases and supplemental oxygen delivered to maintain the arterial pO_2 at greater than 80 mmHg. Blood transfusion may be necessary to provide sufficient hemoglobin to maintain normal oxygen carrying capacity.

Cerebral blood flow is dependent on systemic arterial pressure and arterial pCO_2, especially shortly after head trauma. Normalization of blood pressure and maintenance of pCO_2 at 26 - 28 mmHg is sufficient to maintain adequate cerebral blood flow under most circumstances. Keep in mind that the pCO_2 cannot be allowed to rise too high as it may aggravate intracranial pressure (see 2.a.).

2. Preventing/treating intracranial hypertension

The following types of medical management are suitable only after consultation with the neurosurgeon. They should not be used in routine management without the neurosurgeon's express direction.

The purpose of these treatments is to prevent, control, or diminish intracranial hypertension, regardless of its cause. In addition to mass lesions, acute brain swelling (a vascular engorgement phenomena) and brain edema can complicate any primary brain injury to cause intracranial hypertension.

a. Induced hypocapnia

Arterial carbon dioxide concentration profoundly affects cerebral circulation. When abnormally elevated, cerebrovasodilatation occurs, increasing intracranial blood volume and intracranial pressure. Conversely, reduction of pCO_2 reduces intracranial blood volume and, secondarily, intracranial pressure. Additionally, hyperventilation tends to reduce intracerebral acidosis and increase cerebral metabolism, both of which are beneficial. Therefore, hyperventilation is recommended to reduce arterial pCO_2, maintaining it at 26 to 28 mmHg. This procedure usually requires endotracheal intubation, controlled ventilation, and intermittent iatrogenic paralysis. Intubation should be performed **early** for the comatose patient. Care must be taken to assure that injudicious intubation does not cause further intracranial problems due to increased intracranial pressure elevations from coughing or gagging during intubation.

Hypocapnia can reduce cerebral circulation to the point where cerebral ischemia occurs. Blood gases **must** be monitored closely. **A neurosurgeon should direct deliberate efforts to produce hypocapnia, because this form of treatment can cause complications if not properly monitored.**

b. Fluid control

Intravenous fluids should be administered judiciously to prevent overhydration, which augments cerebral edema. Similarly, intravenous fluid used for maintenance must not be hyposomolar.

c. Diuretics

Diuretics such as mannitol, which cause diuresis by producing intravascular hyperosmolarity, are widely used for severe brain injury. Mannitol undoubtedly can be very effective in shrinking the brain and lowering intracranial pressure. However, other effects may cause major problems. In the emergency department, this agent should be administered **only** with the consent of a neurosurgeon, or to buy time when neurosurgical capabilities will be delayed, and the patient is deteriorating. For the average patient, 1 gm/kg is used. Care must be taken to prevent subcutaneous infiltration. The neurosurgeon may also recommend loop diuretics, such as furosemide, (40 to 80 mg IV for adults). These medications act by medically decompressing the brain, and may buy up to several hours of reduced intracranial pressure. A urinary catheter is required.

d. Steroids

The use of steroids for patients with head injury, although very common in the recent past, has become increasingly controversial. Many neurosurgeons no longer routinely employ steroids in the management of head injury.

VI. Other Manifestations of Head Injury

A. Seizures

Seizures, either full-blown convulsions or focal seizures, can occur with any injury. Seizures are common at the time of injury or shortly thereafter, and do not necessarily portend the development of chronic epilepsy. The neurosurgeon may recommend no treatment. Prolonged or repetitive seizures may be associated with intracranial hemorrhage and should be treated aggressively, because they may cause cerebral hypoxia, brain swelling, and increased intracranial pressure. A common treatment regimen consists of 10 mg diazepam via an intravenous bolus. Respiratory exchange should be closely monitored. If the patient tolerates diazepam and has another convulsion, the dose may be repeated once **with caution**. Diphenylhydantoin, 1 gm IV at a rate of 50 mg/minute, should be started as soon as possible. If the convulsions persist despite diazepam and diphenylhydantoin, the patient should be given phenobarbital or an anesthetic. The injured brain tolerates anesthesia well. The use of diphenylhydantoin is often recommended for severely injured patients as a preventative measure, even if the patient has not had a seizure.

B. Restlessness

Restlessness frequently accompanies brain injury and/or cerebral hypoxia. Its development in a previously quiet patient may be the first clinical expression of an expanding intracranial mass. Restlessness can often be controlled by correcting the cause. Primary attention should be directed to the possibility of cerebral hypoxia and its etiology. A distended bladder, painful bandages, tight casts, or systemic hypoxia may also induce restlessness. Only when these etiological factors have been treated or ruled out is the use of drugs justified to control the restlessness.

The use of narcotics and some sedatives, particularly morphine, is condemned on the premise that they will mask changes in the state of consciousness and other neurological signs. Chlorpromazine, 10 to 25 mg IV, may be helpful for severe agitation. This agent must be administered carefully to avoid hypotension.

C. Hyperthermia

Hyperthermia is disastrous for the patient with an injured brain. Elevations in body temperature increase the rate of brain metabolism and levels of carbon dioxide. The higher the temperature, the greater the risk to the patient.

A head-injured patient with hyperthermia should be placed on a hypothermia blanket, and shivering should be controlled with chlorpromazine.

VII. Scalp Wounds

Despite the dramatic appearance of scalp wounds, they are usually tolerated well and cause few complications. Scalp wounds usually heal well if general principles of good wound management are followed. The location and type of injury to the scalp gives the physician a better understanding of the force and direction of the energy transmitted to the brain.

A. Blood Loss

Blood loss from scalp wounds can be extensive, especially in children. If the adult patient is in shock, bleeding from the scalp alone is usually not the cause. The general principles of scalp wound care include locating and stopping the bleeding. In the case of severed large vessels (ie, superficial temporal arteries), the vessels should be clamped with hemostats and ligated. Moderately severe bleeding from a deep scalp laceration can usually be controlled temporarily by applying direct pressure or placing hemostats on the galea and reflecting them backwards. For the unconscious patient, self-retaining retractors can be used.

B. Inspection of the Scalp Wound

One should inspect the wound carefully and, wearing a sterile glove, palpate inside the laceration for signs of a skull fracture. Depressed skull fractures can usually be palpated, although the presence of a subgaleal hematoma can confuse the findings. Wound inspection also includes looking for cerebrospinal fluid leaks, which may indicate not only a skull fracture, but also an arachnoid and dural tear. A neurosurgeon should be consulted before the wound is closed for all cases involving open fractures or depressed fractures of the skull.

C. Repairing the Scalp Wound

The first step in wound care is to irrigate the scalp wound with copious amounts of saline. Debris, including hair, must be removed. **Do not** remove bone fragments, because they may be tamponading intracranial bleeding. The neurosurgeon should remove bone fragments in the operating room. When in doubt, always consult a neurosurgeon. If transfer to a definitive-care facility is required, definitive surgical closure of a scalp wound can be delayed. However, temporary repair should be done to prevent further contamination of the wound.

When possible, primary definitive repair should be accomplished under sterile technique with meticulous attention to the wound, as **scalp wounds may become infected.** The area immediately around the laceration should be shaved. The galea is closed first, using interrupted sutures. The skin is then sutured and a nonadherent dressing applied. The head wrap, if applied, should be just tight enough to apply mild pressure and prevent subgaleal accumulation of blood.

VIII.Definitive Surgical Management

Within two hours of injury, essential diagnostic studies should be completed. Although meeting this standard is difficult, delay can be extremely costly for the patient. If a neurosurgeon is not available at the facility initially receiving the patient, expeditious transfer of the patient to a hospital with an available neurosurgeon is necessary.

In exceptional circumstances, rapidly expanding intracranial hematomas (usually epidural hematomas) may be imminently life-threatening and may not allow time for transfer if neurosurgical care is some distance away. Although this circumstance is rare in urban settings, it may occur occasionally in rural areas. In such circumstances, emergency burr holes can be considered if a surgeon, properly trained in the procedure, is available.

If definitive neurosurgical care is not immediately available, the purpose of an emergency burr hole is to preserve life by evacuating life-threatening intracranial hematomas. The performance of this procedure may be especially important for patients whose neurologic status rapidly deteriorates, and for patients who do not respond to nonsurgical measures. However and before proceeding with the procedure, the physician must consider the following problems:

1. Not all severely head-injured patients have hematomas.

2. A burr hole, placed as little as 2 mm away from a hematoma, may not locate it.

3. A burr hole itself may cause brain damage or intracranial hemorrhage.

4. Burr-hole evacuation of a hematoma may not be life-saving.

5. A burr hole can consume as much time as getting the patient to a neurosurgeon.

Therefore, unless a neurosurgeon directs otherwise, only a single burr hole is advised. This should be placed **on the side of the largest pupil**, and only in comatose patients with decerebrate or decorticate posturing whose posturing does not respond to endotracheal hyperventilation and dehydrating agents (ie, 1 gm/kg mannitol).

Emergency burr holes should be used only in exceptional circumstances and only with the advice and consent of a neurosurgeon. The indications for a burr hole performed by a nonneurosurgeon are few, and widespread use as a desperation maneuver is not recommended or supported by the Committee on Trauma. The procedure should only be employed if, in the judgment of a neurosurgeon, the burr hole can be performed in a timely manner, and when definitive neurosurgical care cannot be rendered expeditiously. In almost all instances this means that definitive neurosurgical care is many miles or several hours away. The Committee on Trauma strongly recommends that those who anticipate the need for this procedure receive training in the procedure from a neurosurgeon.

IX. Summary

A. Secure and maintain an open airway.

B. Ventilate the patient to maintain oxygenation and to avoid hypercarbia.

C. Treat shock, if present, and look for cause.

D. Except for shock, restrict fluid intake to maintenance levels.

E. Perform a minineurological examination.

F. Establish an initial working diagnosis.

G. Prevent secondary brain injury.

H. Search for associated injuries.

I. Obtain roentgenograms or CT scan as needed, but only after the patient is stable.

J. Consult a neurosurgeon and consider early transfer.

K. Should the patient's condition worsen, consider other diagnoses and forms of treatment; consult with a neurosurgeon, and consider transfer.

L. Continually reassess the patient (neurological examination and Glasgow Coma Scale) to identify changes that necessitate neurosurgical intervention.

Bibliography

1. Anderson DW and McLaurin RL: The National Head and Spinal Cord Injury Survey. **Journal of Neurosurgery** 1980;53:S1-543.

2. Andrews BT, Pitts LH, Lovely MP, et al: Is Computed Tomographic Scanning Necessary in Patients with Tentorial Herniation?: Results of Immediate Surgical Exploration Without Computed Tomography in 100 Patients.**Neurosurgery** 1986;19:408-414.

3. Cooper PR (ed): **Head Injury**, ed 2. Baltimore, Williams and Wilkins, 1987.

4. Gennarelli TA, Spielman GS, Langfitt TW, et al: Influence of the Type of Intracranial Lesion on Outcome from Severe Head Injury: A Multicenter Study Using a New Classification System. **Journal of Neurosurgery** 1982;56:26-32.

5. Gennarelli TA: Emergency Department Management of Head Injuries. **Emergency Medicine Clinics of North America** 1984; 2:749-760.

6. Gildenberg PL, Makela M: Effect of Early Intubation and Ventilation on Outcome Following Head Injury, in **Trauma of the Nervous System**, Dacey RG (ed). Raven, New York, 1985, pp. 79-90.

7. Jennett B, Teasdale G: **Management of Head Injuries**. Philadelphia, Davis, 1981.

8. Masters SJ, McClean PM, Arcarese JS, et al: Skull X-Ray Examinations after Head Trauma: Recommendations by a Multidisciplinary Panel and Validation Study.**New England Journal of Medicine** 1987;316:84-91.

9. Pitts LH: Neurological Evaluation of the Head Injury Patient. **Clinical Neurosurgery** 1982;29:203-224.

10. Seelig JM, Becker DP, Miller JD, et al: Traumatic Acute Subdural Hematoma: Major Mortality Reduction in Comatose Patients Treated Within Four Hours. **New England Journal of Medicine** 1981;304:1511-1518.

**Chapter 6:
Head
Trauma**

Skill Station IX:
Head Trauma Assessment and Management

Equipment

1. Mr. HURT—head trauma manikin

2. Ophthalmoscope

3. Otoscope

4. Table and chairs

5. Semirigid cervical collar

Objectives

1. Performance at this station will allow participants to practice and demonstrate their assessment and diagnostic skills in determining the type and extent of injuries with Mr. HURT (head trauma manikin).

2. Upon completion of this station, the participant will be able to discuss the rationale of clinical signs and symptoms found through assessment.

3. Upon completion of this station, the participant will be able to discuss and establish priorities for initial primary management of the head trauma patient.

4. Participation at this station will allow the student to discuss other diagnostic aids that can be used to determine the area of injury within the brain, and the extent of injury.

**Chapter 6:
Head Trauma**

**Skill
Station
IX**

American College of Surgeons

Head Trauma Assessment and Management

Note: The participant should establish the following in sequence through discussion or demonstration with fellow students and faculty.

I. Primary Survey

A. ABCs.

B. Immobilize and stabilize the cervical spine.

C. Brief neurological examination.

    1. Pupillary response
    2. AVPU

II. Secondary Survey and Management

A. Inspect head.

    1. Lacerations
    2. Nose and ears for presence of cerebrospinal fluid leakage

B. Palpate head.

    1. Fractures
    2. Lacerations for underlying fractures

C. Palpate all scalp lacerations.

    1. Brain tissue
    2. Depressed skull fractures
    3. Debris

D. Perform minineurological exam (Glasgow Coma Scale).

    1. Eye-opening response
    2. Verbal response
    3. Best limb motor response

E. Palpate cervical spine for fractures and apply semirigid cervical collar, if needed.

F. Determine extent of injury.

G. Reassess patient continuously (observe for signs of deterioration)

    1. Frequency
    2. Parameters to be assessed

Index to Mr. HURT Injuries

1. Open, depressed skull fracture on the right

2. Zygomatic fracture (Le Fort III fracture) on the right

3. Maxillary fracture (Le Fort I fracture) on the right

4. Mandibular fracture on the left

5. Nasal fracture

6. Multiple fractures, C-6 vertebra

7. Unequal pupils

8. Hemotympanum on the right

Chapter 7:
Spine and Spinal Cord Trauma

Objectives:

Upon completion of this topic, the physician will be able to identify principles of management, demonstrate the ability to assess spinal trauma, and apply immobilization techniques for patients with vertebral and/or spinal cord injuries.

Specifically, the physician will be able to:

A. Discuss the principles involved in evaluating vertebral and spinal cord trauma.

B. Identify the types of vertebral injuries and outline methods of treatment.

C. Given a simulated patient with suspected cervical vertebral and spinal cord injuries, demonstrate the ability to assess and manage the multiply injured patient.

D. Given a simulated patient with suspected cervical vertebral and spinal cord injuries and appropriate equipment, apply techniques to safely immobilize the neck and spine.

E. Given a series of roentgenograms depicting cervical spine injuries, outline anatomical assessment principles and techniques for detecting abnormalities.

**Chapter 7:
Spine and
Spinal Cord
Trauma**

I. Introduction

The physician must be continually cognizant that injudicious manipulation or movement and inadequate immobilization can cause additional spinal injury and decrease the patient's overall prognosis.

Vertebral injuries may be present without spinal cord injury. However, the potential for cord injury is always present, and careful patient handling is essential. **A vertebral column injury should be presumed and immobilization of the entire patient maintained until screening roentgenograms are obtained and fractures or fracture-dislocations are ruled out.**

II. History of Injury

Knowledge of the patient's neurological condition is very important. A description of how the patient sustained the injury is significant in order to understand the mechanism of injury and potential for further injury. Ambulance personnel can provide valuable information, ie, presence of paralysis immediately postinjury or deterioration of the patient's sensorimotor status. This information is essential to assess and document the site and extent of injury and/or the paralysis present.

Any patient sustaining an injury above the clavicle or a head injury resulting in an unconscious state should be suspected of having an associated cervical spinal column injury. Any injury produced by high-speed vehicles should arouse suspicion of concomitant spine and spinal cord injury.

III. Assessment

A. General

Examination of any suspected case of spinal injury must be carried out with the patient in a neutral position and without any movement of the patient's spine. The neck and trunk must not be flexed, extended, or rotated. The patient should be brought to the emergency department properly immobilized. Although a semirigid cervical collar is useful, securing the head to a spine board and bolster-splinting the neck is equally or more effective. The patient should be left **completely immobilized** until roentgenograms are taken to rule out vertebral fractures.

Total spinal immobilization is the goal. Not only the head and neck, but also the chest, pelvis, and lower extremities must be securely immobilized.

A **conscious** patient with paralysis is usually able to identify pain at the site of injury, because loss of sensation is below this level. **Remember,** paralysis and loss of sensation may mask intra-abdominal and lower-extremity injuries. As the spine is carefully palpated, listen to the patient and watch his face for signs of pain.

If the patient is **unconscious**, and the injury is due to a fall or a vehicular accident, the chance of a cervical spine injury is 5% to 10%. Clinical findings that suggest a cervical cord injury in the unconscious patient include:

1. Flaccid areflexia, especially with flaccid rectal sphincter.
2. Diaphragmatic breathing.
3. Ability to flex, but not extend at the elbow.
4. Grimaces to pain above, but not below the clavicle.
5. Hypotension with bradycardia, especially without hypovolemia.
6. Priapism, an uncommon but characteristic sign.

All information obtained from the neurological examination is carefully documented on the chart for easy identification of any changes. In the paralyzed patient, any movement or sensation at or below the level of the injury is important and may affect the prognosis.

Early consultation with a neurosurgeon and/or orthopedic surgeon is essential.

Specific types of neurologic deficit are important only to establish that an injury is present. Once established, consultation and transfer to an institution with neurosurgical and/or orthopedic capabilities is essential.

Spinal immobilization should be continued until removed by the neurosurgical or orthopedic consultant. This usually occurs when no radiographic abnormality has been documented, and no symptoms or signs relating to the spine or cord exist.

B. Vertebral Assessment

Vertebral injuries usually are associated with local tenderness, and less often, with palpable deformity. Careful palpation of the entire spine from the occiput to sacrum should be done with the patient in a supine position. The physician should assess for pain, tenderness, and a posterior "step-off" deformity. Pain usually will be localized when an injured spine is palpated, but the pain may radiate to the arms, around the chest and abdomen, or into the lower extremities. Other diagnostic signs and symptoms include prominence of spinous processes, local tenderness, pain with attempted motion, edema, ecchymosis, visible deformity, and muscle spasms. The physician should also assess for tracheal tenderness or deviation and retropharyngeal hematoma. The position of the head should be noted for muscle spasm and head tilt. These symptoms also help identify and localize the site of injury.

C. Neurological Assessment of Spinal Cord Injury

The patient is carefully examined for motor strength and weakness, sensory disturbances, reflex changes, and autonomic dysfunction. Autonomic dysfunction is identified by lack of bladder and rectal control, and priapism.

Of the many tracts in the spinal cord, only three can be readily assessed clinically. Each is a paired tract that may be injured on one or both sides of the cord. The **corticospinal tract** controls motor power on the same side of the body and is tested by voluntary muscle contractions or involuntary response to painful stimulus. The **spinothalamic track** or **lateral column** transmits pain and temperature sensation from the opposite side of the body. It is tested by pinch or pin prick. The **posterior columns** carry proprioceptive impulses from the same side of the body and are tested by position sense of the fingers and toes or tuning fork vibration.

No demonstrable sensory or motor function is exhibited with a **complete spinal cord lesion.** This situation is dismal, because the chance of useful recovery is small. **Incomplete spinal cord lesions** differ considerably, because recovery can occur. Therefore, a careful examination to determine the presence of any sensory or motor function is essential.

Superficial (pin-prick) or deep pain discrimination indicates an incomplete lesion and lateral column preservation. Because the sensation of light touch is conveyed in both the lateral and posterior columns, it may be the one sensory modality preserved when all other sensations are absent. Sparing of sensation in the sacral dermatomes may be the only sign of incomplete injury. To assess sacral sparing, gently lift the leg and assess the anal, perianal, and scrotal areas. The evaluation for sacral sparing should include sensory perception and voluntary contraction of the anus.

D. Neurogenic and Spinal Shock

The terms neurogenic and spinal shock are often interchanged. However, most neurosurgeons use the term **neurogenic shock** for the hypotension associated with cervical or high thoracic spinal cord injury. Neurogenic shock results from impairment of the descending sympathetic pathways in the spinal cord, the results of which are loss of vasomotor tone, and loss of sympathetic innervation to the heart. The former causes vasodilatation of visceral and lower extremity vessels, pooling of blood intravascularly, and consequent hypotension. Loss of cardiac sympathetic tone produces bradycardia. Therefore, the combination of hypotension and bradycardia due to neurogenic shock is not due to true hypovolemia. The blood pressure often can be restored by elevating the legs to promote blood return to the heart. Atropine can be used to counteract the bradycardia. Alternately, a gentle sympathomimetic agent, ie, phenylephrine, may have the same effect.

Spinal shock refers to the neurologic condition shortly after spinal cord injury. The "shock" to the injured cord may make it appear completely functionless, even though all areas are not permanently destroyed. This produces flaccidity and loss of reflexes instead of the expected spasticity, hyperactive reflexes, and Babinski signs. Days to weeks later, spinal shock disappears and, in areas where no function has returned, spasticity supersedes the flaccid state.

E. Effect on Other Organ Systems

Hypoventilation due to paralysis of the intercostal muscles will result from an injury involving the lower cervical or the upper thoracic spinal cord. If the upper or the middle cervical spinal cord is injured, the diaphragm will also be paralyzed due to involvement of the C-3 through C-5 spinal cord segments, where the motor nerve cells that innervate the diaphragm (via the phrenic nerve) are located. Abdominal breathing and the use of the respiratory accessory muscles will be evident in both instances.

The inability to feel pain may mask a potentially serious injury elsewhere in the body. Particularly, the presence of spinal shock may prevent manifestation of the usual signs of an acute abdomen.

F. Roentgenograms

Lateral cervical spine and chest roentgenograms should be obtained for every patient sustaining multiple trauma.

1. Cervical spine

Lateral cervical spine roentgenograms should be obtained as soon as life-threatening problems are identified and controlled. **All seven cervical vertebrae must be identified.** The patient's shoulders are routinely pulled down when obtaining the lateral cervical spine film to prevent missing fractures or fracture-dislocations of C-6 and C-7. If all seven cervical vertebrae are not visualized with the lateral roentgenogram, a lateral Swimmer's view of the lower cervical and upper thoracic area is obtained. After adequate demonstration of all seven cervical vertebrae, the physician can obtain a chest film and determine the need for further nonurgent spine roentgenograms. Cervical roentgenograms that can be obtained after the first hour to further evaluate the cervical spine include: anteroposterior, oblique cervical, and open-mouth odontoid roentgenograms. These or more sophisticated studies should be done for any patient with a normal cross-table lateral roentgenogram who is suspected (either by signs and symptoms, or by mechanism of injury) of having cervical injury, because even the best portable films will miss 5% to 15% of the injuries. Tomograms may be necessary to confirm a cervical spine injury and determine its stability. A computed tomography (CT) scan may be needed to determine the presence of bone fragments within the spinal canal. Lateral flexion and extension roentgenograms of the cervical spine may be dangerous and should be done under the direct supervision and control of a knowledgeable physician.

2. Thoracolumbar

Anteroposterior and lateral thoracic films are standard. Oblique thoracic films seldom add further information. Anteroposterior, lateral, and oblique films of the lumbar spine are also obtained if indicated.

IV. Types of Spinal Injuries

A. Fractures and Fracture-Dislocation of the Spine

Roentgenograms should be examined for:

a. Anteroposterior diameter of the spinal canal.
b. Contour and alignment of the vertebral bodies.
c. Displacement of bone fragments into the spinal canal.
d. Linear or comminuted fractures of the laminae, pedicles, or neural arches.
e. Soft-tissue swelling.

1. Cervical spine fractures

Cervical spine injuries may result from any one or a combination of these mechanisms of injury: 1) axial loading, 2) flexion, 3) extension, 4) rotation, 5) lateral bending, and 6) distraction. **Cervical spine injuries resulting in unstable fractures, fracture-dislocations, and/or cord injury require transfer to a definitive-care facility.** When in doubt, consult with a neurosurgeon or orthopedic surgeon.

a. C-1 (Atlas)

A fracture of C-1 (atlas) usually involves a blowout of the ring (Jefferson fracture). The mechanism of injury of a C-1 fracture is usually an axial load. It will appear as a fracture of the lamina on the lateral roentgenogram and is seen best on an open mouth view of the C-1-2 area. **Remember, one third of these fractures are associated with a C-2 fracture.** They are **not** usually associated with cord injuries. However, they are **unstable** and should be treated initially with the application of a semirigid cervical collar, and immobilization of the entire patient on a long spine board.

b. C-2 (Axis)–dislocation of C-2

Injuries to C-2 may displace the odontoid posteriorly into the spinal canal. Odontoid subluxation occurs because of injury to the transverse ligament that attaches the odontoid to the anterior arch of C-1. Bony injury may not occur; therefore this diagnosis should be considered whenever the space between the anterior arch of C-1 and the odontoid is greater than 5 mm. Displacement can occur **without** cord injury due to Steel's "Rule of Three": **one-third of the area in the atlas is occupied by the odontoid, one-third by an intervening space, and one-third by the spinal cord.** Room posterior to the odontoid is thus available for displacement. However, this situation is dangerous because excessive head motion can transect the cord. Head and spine immobilization is critical.

c. C-2 (Axis) - fractures

Three types of fractures may be associated with the odontoid. All can be very difficult to see on routine roentgenograms. If suspected, more views, tomograms, or CT are needed.

1) **Type I** usually occurs above the base of the odontoid and is most often stable.

2) **Type II** occurs at the base of the odontoid and is usually unstable. **Remember,** in children under the age of six, the epiphysis may be present and may appear as a fracture at this level.

3) **Type III** is a fracture of the odontoid that extends into the vertebral body.

Type I can be treated with a semirigid cervical collar or brace. However, all types should be transported to a definitive-care hospital for further evaluation and possible surgical intervention or halo immobilization.

d. Rotary subluxation–odontoid

Rotary subluxation of the odontoid may be seen in relation to the ring of the C-1 vertebra. This injury is diagnosed by an odontoid-view roentgenogram. The odontoid will appear farther from the smaller appearing C-1 segment, relative to the position of the subluxation. This injury is most often seen in children. Treatment of subluxation injuries is usually best managed in a definitive-care facility.

e. Posterior element fractures

The "Hangman's Fracture" (name derived from judicial hangings) involves the posterior elements of C-2. The mechanism of this injury is extension and distraction or extension and axial compression. This is an unstable fracture. Patients with a "Hangman's Fracture" should **not** be placed in cervical traction if the mechanism of injury is secondary to distraction. Such patients should be transferred to a definitive-care facility.

f. C-3 through C-7

Various combinations of fractures and/or fracture-dislocations may be seen in C-3 through C-7. The mechanism of injury in **stable** fractures is usually flexion axial loading, extension axial loading, or flexion rotation injuries.

When examining a lateral c-spine film, assess the distance between the pharynx and the anterior/inferior border of C-3. The soft-tissue prevertebral thickness at this level should be less than 5 mm between the pharynx and vertebral body. An increase in this area of density is indirect evidence of a vertebral fracture, notoriously associated with a minimally displaced C-2 fracture.

Children normally have prevertebral thickness that is two-thirds of the prevertebral thickness of C-2. The distance will vary with inspiration and expiration. When assessing for a hematoma at this level in children, **remember that forced expiration or crying increases the distance between the pharynx and the anterior/inferior border of C-3.**

Below the larynx, the tracheal air shadow is further from the anterior vertebral bodies because of the interposition of the esophagus. The best rule for prevertebral hematoma in this area is that the distance to the air shadow should be less than the width of the vertebral body.

Patients with **unstable** vertebral injuries of C-3 through C-7 require transfer to a definitive-care hospital. Specifically, these patients include those with:

1) An unstable fracture identified by disruption of the anterior and all of the posterior elements.

2) An unstable fracture identified by overriding of a superior vertebra on the adjoining inferior vertebra by more than 3.5 mm.

3) An unstable fracture identified by angulation between two adjoining vertebra greater than 11 degrees.

g. Facet dislocations

Facet dislocations may also produce an **unstable** vertebral injury, especially bilateral facet dislocations. Consider a unilateral facet dislocation if the superior vertebra is displaced on the adjoining inferior vertebra by 25%. Consider a bilateral facet dislocation if displacement is greater than 50%. Malalignment of the cervical spinous processes on an anteroposterior roentgenogram is also suggestive of unilateral facet dislocation.

2. Cervical spinal cord injuries

A bone fleck off the superior aspect of the vertebral body demonstrates an extension-type injury. It is usually stable and does not involve cord damage. The classic tear-drop sign may be seen with a bone chip off the anterior/inferior aspect. Cord injuries are often associated with this radiographic tear-drop finding, an ominous sign that may indicate displacement of the disc or posterior fragment of the vertebral body into the spinal canal.

Spinal cord injuries can occur in the cervical spine with an essentially stable fracture, because the vertebral body collapses and is displaced posteriorly into the cord. These injuries may range from fracture of the body without displacement and cord damage, to severe vertebral disruption with complete paralysis.

3. Thoracic spine fractures T-2 through T-10

Fractures in this region are usually the result of hyperflexion, which produces wedge compression of one or more vertebral bodies. The amount of wedging is usually quite small, and the anterior portion of the vertebral body is rarely more than 25% shorter than the posterior body. Due to the rigidity of the rib cage, most of these fractures are stable. Where the kyphosis exceeds 30 degrees, internal stabilization probably will be required to prevent further deformity. The thoracic spinal canal is narrow in relation to the spinal cord, so that thoracic spinal cord injuries commonly are complete.

4. Thoracolumbar fractures

Fractures at this level are frequently due to the relative immobility of the thoracic spine compared to the lumbar spine. They most often result from a combination of acute hyperflexion and rotation and consequently are commonly unstable. Because the spinal cord terminates and the nerve roots that compose the cauda equina arise at the thoracolumbar junction, an injury at this level will produce bladder and bowel signs (spinal cord) and decreased sensation and movement in the lower extremities (cauda equina) in various combinations.

5. Lumbar fractures

Disruption of the posterior ligaments by an acute hyperflexion injury in the lumbar region will produce an unstable fracture requiring internal stabilization. The neurological signs associated with a lumbar fracture may be similar to those of a thoracolumbar fracture. However, lumbar fracture neurological signs result only from involvement of the cauda equina, which include those nerve roots innervating the bladder.

B. Wounds

The most common of open spinal wounds are those caused either by missile injuries or stabbings. A bullet passing through the vertebral canal usually results in complete neurological deficit. The physician should assess for cerebral spinal fluid drainage from the wound. Hemopneumothorax, acute abdomen, or great vessel injury is often associated with an open spinal injury and takes precedence for treatment.

V. Treatment

A. Immobilization

Prehospital care personnel usually immobilize patients before their transport to the emergency department. Any patient with a suspected spine injury must be immobilized above and below the suspected injury site until injury has been ruled out by roentgenograms. The proper technique for spinal immobilization is outlined in Skill Station X. **Remember,** these protective devices must not be removed until absence of cervical spine injury is documented.

Immobilization with a semirigid collar does not necessarily assure stabilization of the cervical spine. Immobilization to a spine board with sandbags may be more effective in limiting certain neck motions. **Cervical spine injury requires continuous immobilization of the entire patient with a semirigid cervical collar and backboard before and during transfer to a definitive-care facility.**

B. Intravenous Fluids

Intravenous fluids usually are limited to maintenance levels unless specifically needed for the management of shock. Hypovolemic shock can usually be differentiated from neurogenic shock by tachycardia in the former and bradycardia in the latter. If in doubt, elevate the legs, and if the blood pressure does not improve, administer a fluid challenge. Overzealous fluid administration can easily cause pulmonary edema in a spinal cord injury patient. A urinary catheter is inserted to monitor urinary output and prevent bladder distention.

C. Medications

Proper limitation of fluid intake usually obviates the need for diuretics. The value of steroids is controversial; however, they are frequently used in the early management of spinal injuries. Steroids used should be determined in consultation with a neurosurgeon. Ideally, a management protocol is established by consultation.

D. Transfer

Patients with unstable fractures or a documented neurological deficit should be transferred to a definitive-care facility. For physicians who do not routinely see such injuries, the safest procedure is to transfer the patient after phone consultation with a specialist. Avoid unnecessary delay. The patient should be stabilized; necessary splints, backboards, and/or semirigid cervical collar applied; and the patient transferred under medical supervision. **Remember, high cervical spine injuries can result in partial or total loss of respiratory function.** These patients are best managed by maintaining an adequate airway and ventilation. If endotracheal intubation is indicated, the nasal route should be used if possible.

VI. Summary

A. Attend to life-threatening injuries, avoiding any movement of the spinal column.

B. Establish and maintain proper immobilization of the patient until vertebral fractures or spinal cord injuries have been ruled out.

C. Obtain lateral cervical spine roentgenograms as soon as life-threatening injuries are controlled.

D. Documentation of the patient's history and physical examination are of paramount importance to establish a baseline for any changes in the patient's neurological status (ie, ascertaining progress or deterioration of an incomplete lesion).

E. Obtain consultation with a neurosurgeon and/or orthopedic surgeon.

F. Transfer patients with unstable vertebral fractures or spinal cord injury to a definitive-care facility.

Bibliography

1. Apuzzo MLJ, Heiden JS, Weiss MH, et al: Acute Fractures of the Odontoid Process. **Journal of Neurosurgery** 1978;48:85-91.

2. Bohlman HH: Acute Fractures and Dislocations of the Cervical Spine: An Analysis of 300 Hospitalized Patients. **Journal of Bone and Joint Surgery (AM)** 1979;61:1119-1142.

3. Bohlman HH: Current Concepts Review, Treatment of Fractures and Dislocations of the Thoracic and Lumbar Spine. **Journal of Bone and Joint Surgery** January 1985;67-A,1:165-169.

4. Bosch AE, Stauffer ES, and Nickel VL: Incomplete Traumatic Quadriplegia: A Ten-Year Review. **Journal of the American Medical Association** 1971;216:473-478.

5. Denis F: The Three Column Spine and Its Significance in the Classification of Acute Thoracolumbar Spinal Injuries. **Spine** 1983;8:817-831.

6. Durward OJ, Schweigel JF, and Harrison P: Management of Fractures of the Thoracolumbar and Lumbar Spine. **Neurosurgery** 1981;8:555-561.

7. Harris P: **Thoracic and Lumbar Spine and Spinal Cord Injuries**, New York, Springer-Verlag, 1987.

8. Holdsworth F: Fractures, Dislocation, and Fracture-Dislocations of the Spine. **Journal of Bone and Joint Surgery (AM)** 1970;52A:1534-1551.

9. McCall IW, Park WM, and McSweeney T: The Radiological Demonstration of Acute Lower Cervical Injury. **Clinical Radiology** 1973;24:235-240.

10. McMichan JC, Michel L, and Westbrooks PR: Pulmonary Dysfunction Following Traumatic Quadriplegia. **Journal of the American Medical Association** 1980;243:528-531.

11. Moulton RJ and Clifton GL: Injury to the Vertebrae and Spinal Cord, in **Trauma**, Mattox KL, Moore EE and Feliciano DV (eds). Norwalk, Appleton and Lange, 1988, pp 253-269.

12. Podoisky S, et al: Efficacy of Cervical Spine Immobilization Methods. **Journal of Trauma** 1983;23:461.

13. Wagner FC: Management of Acute Spinal Cord Injury. **Surgical Neurology** 1977;7:346-350.

14. Yashon D, Jane JA, and White RJ: Prognosis and Management of Spinal Cord and Cauda Equina Bullet Injuries in 65 Civilians. **Journal of Neurosurgery** 1970;31:163-170.

Chapter 7:
Spine and
Spinal Cord
Trauma

Skill
Station
X

Skill Station X:
Radiographic Identification of
Cervical Spine Injuries

Equipment

1. Cervical spine roentgenograms (available from the ACS Trauma Department–ATLS Division)

2. Identification key to roentgenograms

3. View boxes to display films.

Objectives

1. Upon completion of this station, the participant will be able to identify various cervical spine injuries by using four (4) specific anatomic guidelines for examining a series of cervical spine roentgenograms.

   a. Alignment
   b. Bones
   c. Cartilage
   d. Soft tissue space

2. Given a series of roentgenograms, the participant will be able to:

   a. Diagnose fractures
   b. Delineate associated injuries
   c. Define other areas of possible injury

**Chapter 7:
Spine and
Spinal Cord
Trauma**

**Skill
Station
X**

Skill Procedure

Radiographic Identification of Cervical Spine Injuries

Note: The guidelines outlined below identify areas of the cervical spine that should be assessed when examining a cervical spine film. Each of these areas should be assessed for potential injury when viewing the specific roentgenogram associated with this skill station .

I. Identify Presence of All Seven Cervical Vertebrae

II. Anatomical Assessment

A. Alignment

Identify and assess the four lordotic curves:

1. Anterior vertebral bodies
2. Anterior spinal canal
3. Posterior spinal canal
4. Spinous process tips

B. Bone

Assess for:

1. Vertebral body–contour and axial height
2. Lateral bony mass

   a. Pedicles
   b. Facets
   c. Laminae
   d. Transverse processes

3. Spinous processes

C. Cartilage

Assess for:

1. Intervertebral discs
2. Posterolateral facet joints

D. Soft-Tissue Spaces

Assess for:

1. Prevertebral space
2. Prevertebral fat stripe
3. Space between spinous processes

**Chapter 7:
Spine and
Spinal Cord
Trauma**

**Skill
Station
X**

III. Assessment Guidelines for Detecting Abnormalities

A. Alignment

  1. Vertebral malalignment > 2.7 mm–dislocation
  2. Anteroposterior spinal canal space < 13 mm–spinal cord compression
  3. Angulation of intervertebral space > 11 degrees

B. Bones

  1. Vertebral body
    a. Anterior height < 3 mm posterior height–compression fracture
    b. Oblique lucency: tear-drop fracture

  2. Lack of parallel facets of the lateral mass–possible lateral compression fracture
  3. Lucency through the tip of the spinous process–avulsion fracture
  4. Atlas and axis (C-1 and C-2)
    a. Distance between posterior aspect of C-1 to anterior odontoid process > 3 mm–dislocation
    b. Lucency through the odontoid process of C-2–fracture

C. Soft-Tissue Space

  1. Widening of the prevertebral space > 5 mm–hemorrhage accompanying spinal injury

  2. Obliteration of prevertebral fat stripe–fracture at same level

  3. Widening of space between spinous processes–torn interspinous ligaments and likely spinal canal fracture anteriorly

IV. Review Cervical Spine Films

Identification Key to X-rays

  1. Normal cervical spine
  2. Inadequate cervical spine (normal)
  3. Lateral swimmer's view
  4. Normal cervical spine (six-year-old pediatric patient)
  5. Normal odontoid with superimposition of incisors (NG tube)
  6. Normal odontoid
  7. Fracture of neural arch of C-1 (Jefferson Fracture) (Atlanto-occipital fracture)
  8. Facet fracture of C-1 and C-2 with subluxation
  9. C-4 to C-5 fracture with subluxation
  10. "Hangman's Fracture" (C-2 to C-3 neural arch)
  11. C-5 on C-6 fracture

Skill Station XI:
Immobilization Techniques for Neck and Spinal Trauma

Chapter 7:
Spine and
Spinal Cord
Trauma

Skill
Station
XI

Equipment

1. Live patient model
2. Semirigid cervical collar *
3. Long spine board with straps *
4. Short spine board with straps *
5. Sandbags or similar bolstering devices
6. Straight back chairs for make-shift car seat
7. Blankets for padding
8. Roller-type dressing/bandage
9. Tape

   * Type of equipment used in individual locale

Objectives

1. Upon completion of this station the participant will be able to discuss and/or demonstrate the assessment techniques for examining a patient suspected of having neck and/or spinal injuries.

2. Performance at this station will allow the participant to discuss the principles and techniques for immobilizing the patient with neck and/or spinal injuries.

   a. Seated patient

   b. Supine/prone patient

3. Upon completion of this station the participant will be able to identify when the patient has been properly immobilized in accordance with the techniques and principles outlined during this skill station.

Note: Procedures outlined in this skill station are primarily for demonstration to and information for the physician. These skills may be initially demonstrated by an instructional assistant (EMT-A Instructor), using physician participants as the model and assistants. However, a physician instructor **must** also be present. This skill station can be combined with Skill Station XII–Extremity Immobilization.

**Chapter 7:
Spine and
Spinal Cord
Trauma**

**Skill
Station
XI**

Chapter 7:
Spine and
Spinal Cord
Trauma

Skill
Station
XI

Skills Procedures

Assessment and Immobilization of Neck and Spine Injuries

I. Assessment of Neck and Spine Injuries

A. Assess respiratory status.

    1. Airway patency

        a. Chin lift

        b. Jaw thrust

        c. Intubation (nasotracheal)

    2. Respiratory efforts

B. Assess the patient's level of consciousness.

C. Obtain vital signs.

D. Palpate the cervical spine, noting any abnormality.

    1. Deformity

    2. Grating crepitus

    3. "Boggy" sensation

    4. Increased pain with palpation

E. Assess for spinal pain and location.

F. Assess for paresis and level of paresis.

G. Assess for paresthesia and location/level of paresthesia.

H. Assess for paralysis and site/level of paralysis.

I. Continued reassessment of patient's status.

II. Primary Management: Seated Patient

A. Apply gentle, inline manual immobilization to the patient's cervical spine by placing the hands on either side of the head, gently immobilizing the patient's head and neck in a vertical position.

B. Immobilize the suspected cervical fracture with a semirigid cervical collar.

C. Gently position the short spine board behind the patient.

D. Secure the patient to the board by:

    1. Crossing the shoulder straps across the chest.

Chapter 7:
Spine and
Spinal Cord
Trauma

Skill
Station
XI

2. Applying the leg straps by passing them under the inside, and up and over the outside of the patient's thighs. The straps are placed as close to the groin area as possible.

3. Diagonally attaching the leg straps with the shoulder straps and cinch them up snugly.

4. Placing padding behind the head and neck to provide support between the cervical neck region and the spine board, maintaining a **neutral, vertical alignment of the head and neck.**

5. Securing the patient's head to the board by using cravats, roller bandage, or tape. Wrap it snugly around the patient's forehead and the board. **Do not use the chin strap or any device that might occlude the airway.**

E. Immobilize the patient next on a long spine board.

1. Prepare the long board and place it next to the patient's side.

2. Pivot the patient. (Do **not** use the short board as "handles on the patient," because this causes movement of the spine.)

3. Gently lower the patient on the long spine board, keeping the knees and upper legs bent at right angles to the body until the patient is completely on the long board.

4. Slide the patient onto the backboard and release the leg straps carefully.

5. Lay the patient's legs down and retighten the short board straps.

6. **Secure the entire patient (head, chest, arms, thighs, and lower legs) to the long board with straps.**

III. Primary Management: Supine Patient

A. Prepare the long board with straps.

B. Apply gentle, inline manual immobilization to the head, and apply a semirigid cervical collar.

C. Log-roll the patient as a unit to either side while maintaining inline manual immobilization of the head.

D. Place the long spine board behind the patient.

E. Place padding rolls on the board at the lumbar region, behind the knees, ankles, and neck.

F. Roll the patient as a unit onto the long board and secure with straps across the head, chest, thighs, and lower legs.

IV. Continued Management: Continued Reassessment of the Patient's Status

Chapter 8:
Extremity Trauma

Objectives:

On completion of this topic, the physician will be able to identify life- and limb-threatening musculoskeletal injuries, as well as less serious, but potentially disabling injuries.

The physician also will be able to apply the proper principles of initial evaluation and management of these injuries.

Specifically, the physician will be able to:

A. Identify life- and/or limb-threatening injuries to the extremities.

B. Outline priorities in the assessment of extremity trauma.

C. Explain management of extremity injuries in the emergency department.

D. Demonstrate the ability to assess, assign priorities to, and initially manage injuries on a simulated patient, including application of dressings, splints, and traction splints.

**Chapter 8:
Extremity
Trauma**

I. Introduction

Extremity trauma is rarely life-threatening, but associated injuries can be. Certain injuries and combinations of injuries to the skeleton may be permanently disabling if not properly managed. Therefore, management of the multiply injured patient focuses on the initial management of those injuries that often are associated with other injuries demanding immediate intervention. This chapter emphasizes certain aspects of the initial management, which can have a significant impact on long-term outcome, and discussion of those life- and/or limb- threatening injuries.

Patients with apparent isolated extremity trauma should be managed and assessed in the same manner as multisystem trauma patients. Evaluation of extremity injuries is an integral part of the overall approach to the patient.

A. Primary Survey and Resuscitation

1. Airway with cervical spine control

2. Breathing

3. Circulation with hemorrhage control

4. Disability; brief neurological evaluation

5. Exposure: completely undress the patient

The extremities receive little specific attention during the primary survey–except for direct control of bleeding, which may include maintaining traction on extremities with obvious or suspected fractures, as well as application of direct pressure.

B. Secondary Survey

1. Perfusion

2. Alignment; deformity

3. Function; neurovascular injuries

C. Definitive Care

1. Restoration of perfusion

2. Wound care

3. Restoration of alignment

4. Immobilization by splints or traction

II. Extremity Assessment

Except in cases of obvious, exsanguinating hemorrhage, evaluation of extremity injuries is carried out during the secondary survey.

A. History

The quality of care administered by prehospital and emergency department personnel can significantly affect the recovery and ultimate rehabilitation of any patient with extremity trauma. Information obtained from the patient, relatives, or bystanders at the accident scene should be documented and included as a part of the patient's medical record. Information pertinent to the patient's extremity trauma to consider and inquire about include:

1. Mechanisms of injury

If the patient was injured in **an automobile accident**, inquiries must be made regarding : 1) where the patient was in the vehicle (driver or passenger); 2) whether seat belts were fastened and what type were being worn; 3) whether the patient was ejected from the vehicle; and 4) whether the windshield or dashboard was damaged. Other important information concerning the mechanism of injury includes whether the patient: 1) was a pedestrian; 2) fell from a significant height; 3) was injured as the result of fire, smoke, and/or an explosion; and 4) was injured in an industrial work place, sustaining a crushing injury.

2. Environment

Prehospital care personnel should be queried concerning 1) patient exposure for any length of time to temperature extremes, 2) pavement burns and abrasions, 3) near-drowning complications, 4) contaminating factors such as dirt, animal feces, or fresh water, and 5) whether the patient's clothing was torn or intact.

3. Predisposing factors

Specific predisposing factors that may alter the patient's condition, treatment regimen, and outcome include: 1) ingestion of alcohol and/or drugs; 2) emotional problems or illnesses; 3) underlying medical illnesses; and 4) previous injuries, especially to the same extremity.

4. Findings at the accident site

Findings at the accident site that may help the physician identify potential injuries include: 1) the position in which the patient was found, 2) bleeding or pooling of blood at the scene and the estimated amount, 3) bone or fracture ends that may have been exposed, 4) open wounds in proximity to obvious or suspected fractures, 5) obvious deformity or dislocation, and 6) spontaneous movement of extremities.

5. Prehospital care

Prehospital care must be reported and documented. Care administered that is pertinent to extremity injuries includes: 1) changes in the limb's function, perfusion, or neurologic state; 2) spontaneous reduction of fractures or dislocations accomplished at the scene; 3) dressings and splints applied; 4) extrication procedures; and 5) any delay incurred at the accident site or en route to the hospital.

B. Physical Examination

The patient must be completely undressed for adequate examination. Assessment of extremity injuries should always compare an injured extremity with the uninjured extremity.

1. Look

Visually assess the extremities for 1) color and perfusion; 2) deformities such as angulation or shortening; 3) swelling, discoloration, and bruising; 4) muscle spasm (may not be apparent in the patient with head or spinal cord injuries); and 5) wounds.

2. Feel

The extremities should be assessed for sensation, tenderness, crepitation (feel very carefully and avoid vigorous palpation), pulse (Doppler), capillary filling, and warmth.

3. Movement

Active range of motion should be assessed. Passive range of motion should be assessed cautiously in an extremity suspected of being fractured or dislocated. Neither an extremity with an obvious fracture or dislocation nor an extremity that the patient refuses to move actively should be moved passively.

C. Fracture Assessment

Clinically, fractures are either closed or open. **Any obvious or suspected fracture near a wound should be assumed to be an open fracture, even if the fracture cannot be seen in the wound.**

Open fractures are classified by the extent and complexity of the wound, degree of contamination, and the configuration of the fracture as seen on roentgenograms.

1. Extremity injuries associated with potentially life-threatening complications

Certain extremity injuries are considered life-threatening because of associated complications. Examples include: 1) crush injuries of the abdomen and pelvis, and major pelvic fractures; 2) traumatic amputations of the arm, forearm, thigh, or leg , complete or incomplete; and 3) massive open long-bone fractures with ragged, dirty wounds.

2. Limb-threatening injuries

Limb-threatening injuries include: 1) vascular injuries proximal to the knee or elbow, with or without fractures; 2) crush injuries to an extremity; 3) compartment syndromes; 4) dislocations of the knee or hip; 5) fractures, with or without dislocations, about the elbow or knee; 6) fractures with vascular or nerve injury; and 7) open fractures.

3. Associated fractures or dislocations

Certain musculoskeletal injuries, because of their common mechanism of injury, are often associated with a second injury that may or may not be immediately apparent. Specific examples include:

a. Knee injuries—look for femur fractures, hip dislocations, and pelvic fractures if the patient has been in an automobile accident. In the presence of an ipsilateral femur (or tibia) fracture, a complete examination of the knee is impossible. But the presence of a knee effusion is enough of a clue that a significant knee injury exists.

b. Hyperextension injuries of the wrist—may occur with fractures of the proximal shaft or distal ends of the humerus, or with elbow dislocations, clavicular fractures, and injuries to the hand and forearm.

c. Compression fractures of one or more vertebral bodies, tibial plateau(s), ankles, calcaneal fractures, and femoral fractures may all occur in the patient who has fallen from a height and landed on his feet.

d. Acetabular fractures and posterior dislocations and fracture-dislocations of the hip may occur with ipsilateral fractures of the femur. Roentgenograms of an obvious or suspected fracture of the femur must always include the hip and knee.

e. Bilateral injuries—an obvious injury to one extremity may divert attention from a less obvious injury to another.

f. Pelvic fractures—usually the result of severe trauma, and may accom-pany visceral injuries to the abdomen and genitourinary systems.

4. Occult fractures

Definitive assessment of the multiply injured patient with obvious, life-threatening injuries is a major challenge. Occult fractures may be easily overlooked in such a patient. The following fracture patterns must be specifically considered.

a. In cases of head injury, cervical spine fractures and dislocations—particularly C-6 and C-7—can be overlooked clinically. They also may be missed roentgenographically or misinterpreted on screening roentgenograms because of an overlying shoulder position. Shoulder retraction is necessary, and should be routine in obtaining cervical roentgenograms of the trauma patient. If this method fails to reveal all seven cervical vertebrae, a swimmer's view should be obtained. Visualization of all seven cervical vertebrae should include the C-7 to T-1 interspace, if possible. All injuries above the clavicle imply cervical injury until it has been definitely ruled out.

b. Fractures of the clavicle, scapula, and humerus, as well as dislocations of the glenohumeral joint may be overlooked in patients with associated severe thoracic injury. Conversely, fractures of the scapula may be a clue to an underlying, severe thoracic injury.

c. Nondisplaced fractures of the forearm, femur, or pelvis may be missed because of a thick muscle covering and soft tissue covering. In the absence of an obvious fracture, complex dislocations of the wrist may be missed because of inexperience in interpreting the roentgenograms.

D. Blood Loss Assessment

1. Closed injury

Closed extremity injuries may produce enough blood loss to cause hypovolemic shock. Patients with multiple closed fractures, particularly those of the femur and pelvis, are at greater risk. The bleeding may go undetected because it is sequestered in the extremity or retroperitoneal space.

Fractures of the pelvis may cause hypovolemic shock with the loss of six or more units of blood. Closed fractures of the femur may lose two to three units into the thigh. However, fractures should not automatically be assumed to be the cause of hypovolemic shock in trauma patients. Other factors, such as abdominal injuries, should be assumed to be the cause of bleeding until ruled out.

2. Open injury

Open fractures result in blood loss that begins at the time and site of the injury; thus the physician may be unable to calculate or appreciate the degree of prehospital blood loss. Obtaining an accurate history and carefully monitoring the patient's blood volume will assist in assessing the degree of blood loss. As a rule, blood loss from open fractures is far greater than estimated.

E. Dislocation and Fracture-Dislocation Assessment

It is usually not possible, on clinical examination, to differentiate between dislocations and fracture-dislocations of a joint. Only roentgenographic evaluation will distinguish between these types of injuries.

Dislocation, particularly of major joints, may produce neurovascular injury that can result in permanent impairment or a limb-threatening condition. Allowing a major joint to remain dislocated for a protracted period of time can result in both accentuated traction injury to the nerve, and/or irreversible muscle damage due to vascular compromise. The neurovascular bundles are particularly vulnerable about the knee, elbow, and ankle. Prolonged delay in reduction of a dislocated hip increases the chances of aseptic necrosis of the femoral head and permanent disability.

All dislocations, even of small joints, are painful injuries. They cannot be easily splinted, and pain cannot be relieved until the dislocation is reduced.

F. Assessment of Neurovascular Bundle Injury

Nerves and vessels run together in bundles in the forearm, leg, hand, and foot. Local swelling, vessel disruption, or contained hemorrhage can produce injury to vessels and nerves in the extremity. Penetrating injury to the extremity, particularly missile-type wounds, may disrupt the solid bone structures and muscles, while sparing the more elastic structures, such as vessels and nerves. However, all structures may be injured. Assessment of neurovascular status is the first step in evaluation of extremity injuries.

1. Vascular injuries

Vascular injuries disrupt the integrity of the vessel wall, with bleeding or thrombosis resulting in impairment of distal circulation and ischemia. Brisk bleeding from the depths of a wound suggests a vascular injury. It is notable that complete tears of an artery may produce less bleeding than partial tears due to the contractility of the vessel. Arterial and venous injuries due to partial tears are likely to bleed for a prolonged period of time. A large hematoma or injuries to the neural structures anatomically associated with the vessels, also suggest a significant vascular injury.

Examination of distal pulses is crucial. The mere presence of pulses does not rule out vascular injury. Any abnormality of distal pulses strongly suggests a vascular injury and must be explained. **Diminished pulses or pallor of the skin should not be attributed to spasm. Extremity pulses should be evaluated to assure that the blood supply to the extremity has not been compromised.**

Although measures of pressure and Doppler examination are useful in evaluating extremity perfusion, **angiograms provide the best definitive evaluation of a suspected vascular injury when the diagnosis is in doubt.** Roentgenograms and angiograms should **not** be done until the patient's condition is stabilized and the injured extremity is evaluated, dressed, and splinted.

2. Nerve injuries

Nerve injuries may be present as an actual division of the nerve or a physiological disruption. This differentiation usually cannot be made clinically. Physiological nerve disruption usually occurs in closed injuries unless the nerve is anatomically divided by bony fragments. Shock waves created by missiles, or stretching or compression of the nerve fibers may cause variable degrees of paralysis, ranging from partial and temporary to complete and permanent. In general, stretch injuries have a poor prognosis compared with compression injuries.

G. Vascular Impairment

These signs suggest a vascular injury: 1) bleeding, 2) expanding hematoma, 3) bruit, 4) abnormal pulses, 5) impaired distal circulation, 6) decreased sensation, and 7) increasing pain.

Some vascular injuries, such as arterial intimal tears, may not be immediately apparent. Capillary refill may be normal, and the distal pulses may be minimally changed. These injuries may be difficult to identify in the first hour, particularly if there is no obvious bleeding and perfusion of the extremity appears adequate. Reassessment must be done frequently.

In contrast, vascular injuries associated with impaired circulation represent an immediate or potential threat to limb viability and must be recognized and managed promptly. In the patient who is hemodynamically stable, pulse discrepancies, pallor, paresthesia, hypoesthesia and/or any abnormality of motor function suggest possible impairment of nutritional blood flow to the extremity. If any of these abnormalities (particularly any change in pulse) persist after aligning and immobilizing the extremity, a careful investigation for possible vascular injury should be undertaken. With all cases of suspected vascular injury the physician should: 1) check the immobilization device, 2) assess the fracture alignment, 3) reassess distal perfusion, 4) consider a compartment syndrome, and 5) obtain surgical consultation.

If a traction device has been applied to an injured extremity with vascular impairment, the status of the traction must be assessed and any necessary adjustments made. Failure to fully align a long-bone fracture with insufficient traction, or stretching an extremity through excessive traction can result in vascular impairment. If a circular dressing, splint, or cast has been applied, assess for constriction. Release the device if there is any suspicion of it being too tight.

When an arterial injury is suspected, consider early arteriography. The presence of pulses by Doppler examination does not rule out arterial injury. For some patients with obvious and complete arterial occlusion, prompt surgical consultation is mandatory; and surgical exploration may be considered without waiting for an arteriogram.

The classic picture of late, complete extremity ischemia–pain, pallor, pulselessness, paresthesia, and paralysis–indicates profound ischemia. This late manifestation of severe ischemia indicates a surgical emergency, with little time remaining to salvage the extremity. **The goal of management is to identify vascular injuries before full-blown ischemia develops.**

H. Compartment Syndrome

Whenever interstitial tissue pressure rises above that of the capillary bed, local ischemia of nerve and muscle occurs. Permanent paralysis and/or necrosis may result in the form of Volkmann's ischemic contracture, or frank gangrene.

Elevated tissue pressures typically develop within one or more fascial compartments of the leg or forearm. Prompt recognition of a compartment syndrome is essential so that a fasciotomy can be done to release tight muscle compartments, thereby lowering interstitial pressure, before necrosis occurs.

Compartment syndromes usually develop over a period of several hours. They may be initiated by crush injuries, closed or open fractures, sustained compression of an extremity in a comatose patient, or after restoration of blood flow to a previously ischemic extremity. The pneumatic antishock garment may be associated with compartment syndrome, particularly if applied over an injured leg or legs and left inflated for prolonged periods of time. Prolonged application of the PASG on an **uninjured** extremity may also produce a compartment syndrome.

The signs and symptoms of compartment syndrome are: 1) pain, typically increased by passively stretching involved muscles; 2) decreased sensation of nerves within the involved compartment; 3) tense swelling of the involved region; and 4) weakness or paralysis of involved muscles. Distal pulses and capillary filling do not reliably identify compartment syndromes, because they may be intact until late in the evolution of a compartment syndrome, after irreversible changes have occurred. Intracompartmental pressure measurement may help diagnose a suspected compartment syndrome.

I. Amputation

Amputation is a catastrophic extremity injury. Recent techniques allow replantation and functional restoration of the part in certain instances.

The techniques and equipment for replantation are highly sophisticated, and usually are found only in specialized replantation centers. Patients with amputation injuries require rapid assessment and consultation with a specialized center. The surgeon at the definitive-care facility who will be treating the patient decides whether or not the patient is a candidate for replantation.

If the patient is a candidate for replantation, the amputated part should be carefully preserved, and rapidly transported **with the patient** to the replantation center. Time is of the essence. An amputated part will remain viable for only four to six hours at room temperature, or up to 18 hours if cooled. The amputated part should be cleansed of any gross dirt or debris; wrapped in a sterile towel moistened with sterile saline; placed in a sterile, sealed plastic bag; and transported in an insulated cooling chest filled with crushed ice and water. **Do not** allow the amputated part to freeze, **do not** place it in dry ice, and make certain that the amputated part accompanies the patient.

If the patient is not a replantation candidate, consider saving some of the amputated part for grafts on other injured parts of the body. The treating surgeons will make the final decision whether to use such parts.

III. Extremity Trauma Management

Life-threatening problems, ie, airway, breathing, and circulation, are managed first. After these emergencies are controlled, attention can be directed at the specific extremity injury, usually in the definitive-care phase. Patients with extremity injuries are potential candidates for operation, and must not receive anything by mouth.

A. Fractures

1. Open wounds

Any wound associated with a fracture must be managed as if it were an open fracture. The most important factor in successful management of an open fracture is to prevent infection. The management of an open fracture is the management of the wound. Time is of the essence in preventing infection. Open fractures should be definitively treated before eight hours have elapsed from the time of injury. These injuries require consultation and transfer to a facility that has an orthopedic surgeon.

Primary care involves the removal of gross contamination from the wound and the prevention of further contamination. Prehospital personnel should be questioned about the presence of protruding bone and the type and degree of contamination. Open fractures should be aligned with proper splinting techniques. Cover the wound with a dry, sterile dressing. Align and splint the extremity, reinforcing the dressing as necessary. Initiate appropriate antibiotic coverage and administer tetanus prophylaxis.

2. Immobilization

Any fracture or suspected fracture must be immobilized to control pain and prevent further injury. Severely angulated fractures should be aligned.

Distal pulses, skin color, temperature, and neurologic status are assessed before and after aligning. Gentle traction , as an adjunct to splinting and to facilitate alignment, is beneficial when immobilizing long-bone fractures. If possible, the splints should extend one joint above and below the fracture site. For dislocation, immobilize the bone above and below the joint. Roentgenograms, including arteriograms, should **not** be obtained until the extremity is dressed and splinted.

B. Joint Injuries

Management of dislocations and fracture-dislocations has a high priority. **Knee** (tibio-femoral) dislocations, while rare, frequently result in popliteal artery and/or nerve injuries. Dislocations of the **ankle,** which almost invariably involve fractures, may result in skin pressure and necrosis. Dislocations about the **elbow** may clinically resemble supracondylar fractures of the humerus. Shoulder dislocations may have brachial plexus injuries. All dislocations are painful.

Prompt orthopedic consultation should be obtained for all dislocations and fractures. Occasionally, the orthopedic consultant will recommend immediate reduction of a dislocated knee or ankle, especially if his examination of the patient will be delayed. However, reduction of a dislocation should not be attempted without first consulting with the orthopedic surgeon. All dislocations should be reduced as rapidly as possible. Hip or elbow dislocations sometimes require general anesthesia for reduction. The extremity should be supported on pillows or sandbags while the patient awaits definitive care.

C. Open Wounds

Open wounds are best covered with dry, sterile dressings before definitive management. Bleeding is controlled by direct pressure dressings. In rare instances, anatomical pressure points can be used for proximal arterial occlusion to augment hemorrhage control until definitive treatment can be instituted. Prior to surgical management, probing and clamping vessels in the emergency department are unwise procedures. These procedures are difficult, and may endanger associated nerve bundles and increase the risk of infection. Tourniquets should be used only to control hemorrhage from hopelessly injured extremities.

D. Compartment Syndrome

When symptoms or suspicion of a compartment syndrome are present, all potentially constricting materials, ie, circumferential dressings, casts, etc, must be released. If symptoms do not respond rapidly with external decompression, prompt fasciotomy may be required unless compartment pressure measurements definitively rule out compartment syndrome. Pressures over 30 mmHg are considered abnormal. If capabilities for such a procedure are not available locally, immediate orthopedic consultation is advisable, and early transfer is indicated.

E. Antibiotics

Broad-spectrum antibiotics, directed toward the most likely contaminant, should be administered intravenously as soon after the injury as possible. Proper surgical care is the mainstay of wound care. Cultures may be obtained in the emergency department, and should be obtained routinely at the time of wound debridement.

F. Pain Control

Analgesics should be used sparingly, if at all. Immobilization of fractures is the safest and most effective method of pain control. If administered, analgesics should be given intravenously. Intramuscular analgesics should **not** be administered during the initial assessment and treatment phases, especially if the trauma victim is suffering from shock. As circulation in the extremities improves, the patient, emerging from shock, will receive a large dose of analgesics stored in the muscles during the absence of circulation. If a painful procedure must be carried out, such as reduction of a dislocated shoulder, small amounts of analgesic or relaxant, carefully monitored, may be necessary. A 50-50 mixture of oxygen and nitrous oxide may be used as a gas analgesic, especially for pain control during long-distance transfers.

Increasing pain after adequate immobilization raises the possibility of ischemic injury and/or compartment syndrome.

G. Tetanus Immunization

Attention must be directed to adequate tetanus prophylaxis in the multiply injured patient, particularly if open extremity trauma is present. Tetanus immunization depends upon the patient's previous immunization status and the tetanus-prone nature of the wound. (See Appendix C—Tetanus Immunization.)

Table 1
Tetanus Immunization Schedule

Td: Tetanus and diphtheria toxoids adsorbed—for adult use;
TIG: Tetanus immune globulin—human

History of Adsorbed Tetanus Toxoid (doses)	Nontetanus-prone Wounds		Tetanus-prone Wounds	
	Td[1]	TIG	Td[1]	TIG
Unknown or ≤ three	Yes	No	Yes	Yes
≥ three[2]	No[3]	No	No[4]	No

Key to Table 1

[1] For children under 7 years old: DTP (DT, if pertussis vaccine is contraindicated) is preferred to tetanus toxoid alone. For persons 7 years old and older, Td is preferred to tetanus toxoid alone.

[2] If only three doses of fluid toxoid have been received, a fourth dose of toxoid, preferably an adsorbed toxoid, should be given.

[3] Yes, if more than 10 years since last dose.

[4] Yes, if more than 5 years since last dose. (More frequent boosters are not needed and can accentuate side effects.)

IV. Immobilization

Although splinting of extremity injuries must be deferred until the life-threatening injuries have been controlled, all such injuries must be splinted before patient transport. Specific types of splints can be applied for specific fracture needs. The pneumatic antishock garment (PASG) has not proved to be an effective splint for extremity injuries and may be hazardous in fractures of the tibia, particularly open fractures. The PASG should be used only for those patients with blunt abdominal trauma who are in danger of exsanguination from intraperitoneal or retroperitoneal bleeding. The PASG can be used to immobilize lower extremity fractures in patients whose injuries are complicated by shock, and who have femoral or pelvic fractures. All trauma patients should be on a long spine board, which serves as a total body splint. It also eases the multiple transfers required for many transfer patients.

A. Leg and Arm Fractures

The **hand** should be splinted in an anatomic, functional position, with the wrist slightly dorsiflexed and the fingers slightly flexed at all joints. This position can usually be achieved by gently immobilizing the hand over a large roll of gauze.

The **forearm and wrist** are immobilized flat on padded or pillow splints.

The **elbow** is splinted in a flexed position, either by using padded splints or by directly immobilizing to the body with a sling and swath device.

The **arm** is immobilized by splinting to the body or simple application of a sling or swath, which can be augmented with splints for unstable fractures.

Circumferential bandages, used to apply molded and padded splints, can have a tourniquet effect. The extremity must be monitored frequently for vascular compromise. All splints must be padded over bony prominences.

All jewelry, including rings, bracelets, etc, must be removed before splinting any upper extremity injury to prevent pressure on the area and circulatory embarrassment.

B. Femoral Fractures

Femoral fractures are best splinted with traction splints. The traction splint's force is applied distally to the foot, while proximally, the splint is secured to the thigh and hip area. Traction splints may be used for ipsilateral femoral and tibial fractures. Excess traction may cause skin avulsion of the foot, perineal injury, and neurovascular compromise from stretching of anatomic structures.

C. Tibia Fractures

Tibia fractures are best immobilized with a padded board splint or aluminum gutter splint. When aligning a tibial fracture in a splint, make sure the rotation of the fracture is correct, and that the second toe is aligned with the tibial tubercle.

C. Ankle Fractures

Ankle fractures may be immobilized with a pillow splint or padded board splint, avoiding pressure over bony prominences. Assess the neurovascular status before and after the splint is applied.

IV. Summary

The initial assessment and management of extremity trauma are part of the secondary survey in the management of the multiply injured patient. Life-threatening situations must be properly assessed and managed before attention is directed to the injured extremity. The extremity can sustain a variety of injuries, from sprains and fractures to traumatic amputation. A knowledge of the mechanism of injury and history of the accident will enable the physician to diagnose and properly manage the injured extremity. Early alignment of fractures and dislocations and proper splinting techniques can prevent serious complications and late sequelae of extremity trauma. In addition, an acute awareness of the patient's tetanus status, particularly in cases of open fractures, can prevent serious complication. The astute physician, armed with the proper knowledge and skills, can initially and satisfactorily manage most extremity trauma.

In the multiply injured patient with extremity trauma, urgent operative fixation of fractures within the first 24 hours, may reduce mortality and morbidity. It is essential to obtain orthopedic consultation early in the patient's management.

Bibliography

1. American Academy of Orthopaedic Surgeons: **Emergency Care and Transportation of the Sick and Injured**, ed 4. Chicago, 1986, chapters 14-16.

2. American College of Surgeons Committee on Trauma: **Early Care of the Injured Patient**, ed 3. Philadelphia, WB Saunders Co,1982.

3. American College of Surgeons Committee on Trauma: **Guide to Initial Therapy of Soft Tissue Wounds** (reprint). Chicago, American College of Surgeons, 1983.

4. American College of Surgeons Committee on Trauma: **Guide to Prophylaxis Against Tetanus in Wound Management** (reprint). Chicago, American College of Surgeons, 1987.

5. American College of Surgeons Committee on Trauma: Appendix C—Interhospital Transfer of the Injured Patient. **Hospital and Prehospital Resources for Optimal Care of the Injured Patient**, Chicago, American College of Surgeons, 1987.

6. Connolly JF: **The Management of Fractures and Dislocations**, ed 3. Philadelphia, Saunders Co, 1981.

7. Crenshaw AH, ed: **Campbell's Operative Orthopaedics**, ed. 7. St. Louis, CV Mosby Co, 1987.

8. Mubarak SJ, Hages AR: Compartment Syndrome/Volkmann's Contracture in **Management in Orthopedics**, vol 6. Philadelphia, Saunders Co., 1981.

9. Perry MD: **Management of Acute Vascular Injury**, Baltimore, William and Watkins Co, 1981, Chapter 2.

10. Rockwood CA, Green DP: **Fractures,** ed 2. Philadelphia, JP Lippincott Co., 1984.

11. Rosenthal RE: Emergency Department Evaluation of Musculoskeletal Injuries. **Emergency Medicine Clinics of North America** 1984;2:219-244.

**Chapter 8:
Extremity
Trauma**

Chapter 8:
Extremity
Trauma

Skill
Station
XII

Skill Station XII:
Immobilization Techniques
for Extremity Trauma

Equipment

1. Live patient model

2. Assorted extremity immobilization splints, eg, molded, cardboard, or pneumatic (demonstration purposes only)*

3. Leg traction splint*

4. Blanket

   * Devices used by local prehospital personnel

Objectives

1. Upon completion of this station the participant will be able to identify the major neurovascular structures of the upper and lower extremities.

2. Upon completion of this station the participant will be able to discuss the principles and techniques associated with immobilizing extremity injuries.

3. Upon completion of this station the participant will be able to identify when the patient's injured extremity has been properly immobilized in accordance with techniques outlined in this skill station.

Chapter 8:
Extremity
Trauma

Skill
Station
XII

Skill Procedure

Chapter 8:
Extremity
Trauma

Skill
Station
XII

Principles and Techniques of Immobilization for Extremity Trauma

Goal of Splinting: Prevent further injury and control pain.

I. Principles of Extremity Immobilization

A. Assess ABCs and treat life-threatening situations first.

B. Identify neurovascular structures in the injured extremity which may have been compromised as a result of the injury.

C. Select the appropriate size and type of splint for the injured extremity. The device should extend one joint above and one joint below the fractured site.

D. Dress any open wounds.

E. Remove and/or cut open all clothing on the extremity. Remove watches, rings, bracelets, and potentially constricting devices.

F Assess the neurovascular status of the extremity before applying the splint.

G. Apply padding over bony prominences which will be covered by the splint.

H. Apply gentle distal and proximal traction to the extremity before and during application of the splint. Gentle traction should be maintained until the splinting device is secured.

I. Continue to monitor the neurovascular status of the injured extremity.

J. Severely angulated fractures should be aligned.

K. Obtain orthopedic consultation, especially for fracture-dislocations of the joints.

II. Application of the Leg Traction Splint

A. One person should handle the injured extremity, and another should handle the application of the splint.

B. Measure the **unaffected** leg with the traction splint.

　　1. The upper cushioned ring should be placed right under the buttocks and adjacent to the ischial tuberosity.

　　2. Two support straps should be above the knee and two below the knee.

**Chapter 8:
Extremity
Trauma**

**Skill
Station
XII**

C. Cut away clothing (including all foot wear) to expose the injured site. Dress open wounds.

D. The first assistant supports the leg, while the second assistant removes the shoe and sock to assess distal circulation and pedal pulses.

E. The first assistant applies manual traction to the leg, while maintaining support under the fracture and the calf.

F. Reassess distal pulse after applying manual traction.

G. While the first assistant maintains manual traction on the leg, the second assistant applies the ankle hitch around the patient's ankle and upper foot. The bottom strap should be the same length or preferably shorter than the two upper cross straps.

H. Gently lift the fractured limb, while maintaining support and traction. Slide the splint under the affected leg, placing the padded upper ring snugly against the ischial tuberosity.

I. Gently lay the leg on the splint, and extend the leg elevator. Snugly attach the top strap first.

J. While continuing to support the leg and maintain traction, attach the ankle hitch to the traction hook.

K. Apply traction gently to the leg by turning the windlass knob until the extremity appears stable, or in the conscious patient, until pain and spasm are relieved.

L. Reassess the distal, pedal pulses.

M. Secure the remaining straps, making sure they are not too tight.

N. Continually reassess the circulation to the affected limb.

Chapter 9:
Injuries Due to Burns and Cold

Objectives:

Upon completion of this topic, the physician will be able to identify methods of assessment and outline measures to stabilize, manage, and transfer patients with burns and cold injuries.

Specifically, the physician will be able to:

A. Estimate the burn size and determine presence of associated injuries.

B. Outline measures of initial stabilization and treatment of patients with burns, and patients with cold injury.

C. Outline criteria for the transfer of burn patients.

D. Identify special problems and methods of treatment of burn patients, and patients with cold injury.

**Chapter 9:
Injuries Due
to Burns
and Cold**

I. Introduction

Burn and cold injuries constitute a major cause of morbidity and mortality in traumatized patients. Attention to basic principles of initial trauma resuscitation and the timely application of simple emergency measures should minimize the morbidity and mortality in these injuries.

These principles include a high index of suspicion for the presence of airway compromise in smoke inhalation, the maintenance of hemodynamic stability, and fluid and electrolyte balance. The physician also must have an awareness of measures to be instituted for prevention and treatment of the potential complications of thermal injuries, eg, rhabdomyolysis and cardiac dysrhythmias, as seen in electrical burns. Removal from the injury-provoking environment, cautious temperature control, and observation for definite demarcation of nonviable tissue before major debridement also constitute major principles of thermal injury management.

II. Immediate Life-saving Measures for Burn Injuries

A. Airway Distress

Although the larynx protects the subglottic airway from direct thermal injury, the supraglottic airway is extremely susceptible to obstruction as a result of exposure to superheated air. Signs of airway obstruction may not be immediately obvious, although some will warn the examiner of potential airway obstruction. When a patient is admitted after sustaining a burn injury, the physician should be alert to the possibility of airway involvement, identify signs of distress, and initiate supportive measures. Clinical indications of inhalation injury include:

1. Facial burns.

2. Singeing of the eyebrows and nasal hair.

3. Carbon deposits and acute inflammatory changes in the oropharynx.

4. Carbonaceous sputum.

5. History of impaired mentation and/or confinement in a burning environment.

The presence of any of these findings suggests acute inhalation injury. Such injury requires immediate and definitive care, including airway support with endotracheal intubation, and consideration of or early transfer to a burn unit.

B. Stop the Burning Process

All clothing should be removed to stop the burning process. Synthetic fabrics ignite, burn rapidly at high temperatures, and melt into hot plastic residue that continues to burn the patient.

C. Intravenous Lines

After establishing airway patency and identifying and treating immediately life-threatening injuries, intravenous access must be established. Any patient with burns over more than 20% of the body surface area needs circulatory volume support. A large-caliber (at least #16-gauge catheter) intravenous line must be established immediately. The catheter should be placed in a large-caliber peripheral vein. Overlying burned skin should not deter placement of the catheter in an accessible vein. The upper extremities, even if burned, are preferable to the lower extremities because of the high incidence of phlebitis and septic phlebitis in the saphenous veins. Begin infusion with Ringer's lactate solution. Guidelines for establishing the flow rate of Ringer's lactate solution are outlined later in this chapter.

III. Assessing the Burn Injury

A. History

A brief history of the nature of the injury may prove extremely valuable in the management of the burn patient. For instance, serious injuries may be sustained while the victim attempts to escape from the source of the burn. Water-heater explosions, propane gas explosions, and other explosive burns frequently throw the patient some distance, and may result in internal injuries and fractures, ie, myocardial and pulmonary contusions and flail chest. It is essential that the time of the burn be established.

The history, from the patient or relative, should include a brief survey of associated illnesses–including diabetes; hypertension; cardiac, pulmonary or renal disease; and drug therapy. Allergies and sensitivities are also important. The patient's tetanus immunization status should also be ascertained.

B. Body Surface Area

The "Rule of Nines" is a useful and practical guide to determine the extent of the burn. The adult body configuration is divided into anatomic regions that represent 9%, or a multiple of 9%, of the total body surface. Body surface area differs considerably for children. The infant's or young child's head represents a larger proportion of the body surface area, and the lower extremities a lesser proportion, than an adult's. The percentage of total body surface of the infant's head is twice that of the normal adult. **Remember: one surface of the patient's hand represents approximately 1% of his body surface.** This guideline helps estimate the extent of burns of irregular outline or distribution.

C. Depth of Burn

The depth of burn is important in evaluating the severity of the burn, planning for wound care, and predicting functional and cosmetic results. **First-degree burns** are characterized by erythema, pain, and the absence of blisters.

Second-degree burns or partial-thickness burns are characterized by a red or mottled appearance with associated swelling and blister formation. The surface may have a weeping, wet appearance and is painfully hypersensitive, even to air currents.

The full-thickness or third-degree burn appears dark and leathery. The skin may also appear translucent, mottled, or waxy white. The surface is painless and generally dry, but may also be moist. (See Figure 1 at the conclusion of this chapter.)

IV. Stabilizing the Burn Patient

A. Physical Examination

The following must be done in order to plan and direct management of the patient.

1. Estimate extent and depth of burn.

2. Weigh the patient.

3. Assess for associated injuries.

B. Airway

Objective signs of airway injury or history of confinement in a burning environment dictates evaluation of the airway and definitive management. Pharyngeal thermal injuries may produce marked upper airway edema, and early maintenance of the airway is important. The clinical manifestations of inhalation thermal injury may be subtle and frequently do not appear in the first 24 hours. If the physician waits for radiographic evidence of pulmonary injury or change in blood gases, intubation may be not only late, but more difficult because of airway edema.

Major concerns regarding the respiratory status in the patient exposed to smoke and heat are:

1. Inhalation of products of incomplete combustion (carbon particles) and toxic fumes, leading to chemical tracheobronchitis and pneumonia.

2. Direct thermal injury, producing airway mucosal sloughing, bronchorrhea and pulmonary edema.

Always assume carbon monoxide (CO) exposure in patients sustaining burns in enclosed areas. Diagnosis of carbon monoxide poisoning is made primarily from a history of exposure and measurement of carboxyhemoglobin level, if available. The observation of a cherry-red skin color may be an inconstant sign. Headache, nausea, vomiting, and mental disturbances occur at higher carbon monoxide levels. Because of the increased affinity of carbon monoxide for hemoglobin (240 times that of oxygen), it displaces oxygen from the hemoglobin molecule and shifts the oxyhemoglobin dissociation curve to the left. Carbon monoxide dissociates very slowly, and its half-life is 250 minutes while the patient is breathing room air, compared to 40 minutes on 100% oxygen. Therefore, patients exposed to carbon monoxide initially should be placed on 100% O_2.

Early management of inhalation injuries includes endotracheal intubation and mechanical ventilation. Arterial blood gases should be obtained immediately as a baseline for the evaluation of the pulmonary status. However, measurements of arterial pO_2 do not reliably predict carbon monoxide poisoning, because a carbon monoxide partial pressure of only 1 mmHg results in a carboxyhemoglobin level of 40% or greater. Therefore, baseline carboxyhemoglobin levels should be obtained, if possible, and 100% O_2 should be administered when carbon monoxide poisoning is suspected.

C. Circulating Blood Volume

Evaluation of the circulating blood volume is often difficult in the severely burned patient. Blood pressure may be difficult to obtain and is unreliable if measured in a progressively swelling limb. Monitoring hourly urinary outputs reliably assesses circulating blood volume. Therefore, an indwelling urethral catheter should be inserted. A good rule of thumb is to infuse fluids at a rate sufficient to produce 0.7 to 1.0 ml of urine/kilogram body weight/hour for children who weigh 30 kg or less, and 30 to 50 ml per hour in the adult.

The burn patient requires 2 to 4 ml of electrolyte-containing solution/kilogram body weight/percent body surface burn in the first 24 hours to maintain an adequate circulating blood volume and provide adequate renal output. The estimated fluid volume is then proportioned in the following manner: one half of the total estimated fluid is provided in the first eight hours postburn, and the remaining one half in the next 16 hours. **This amount of fluid is required in addition to the patient's daily fluid requirements.**

Any resuscitation formula provides only an estimate. Fluid requirement calculations for infusion rates are based on the **time from injury,** not from the time fluid resuscitation was initiated. The amount of fluid given should be adjusted according to the individual patient's response, ie, urinary output, vital signs, and general condition.

D. Flow Sheet

A flow sheet, outlining the patient's management, should be initiated from the time the patient is admitted to the emergency department. This flow sheet should accompany the patient when he is transferred to the burn unit.

E. Baseline Determination for the Major Burn Patient

1. Blood

Obtain blood samples for CBC, type and crossmatch, carboxyhemoglobin, chemistry profile, and electrolytes. Arterial blood samples should also be obtained for blood gas determinations.

2. Roentgenograms

A chest film should be obtained. An additional film will be required after intubation, and after subclavian or internal jugular vein catheterization is accomplished. Other roentgenograms may be indicated for appraisal of associated injuries.

F. Circumferential Extremity Burns—Maintenance of Peripheral Circulation

1. Remove rings and bracelets.

2. Assess the status of distal circulation, checking for cyanosis, impaired capillary refilling, or progressive neurological signs (ie, paresthesia and deep tissue pain). Assessment is best determined by a Doppler Ultrasonic Meter.

3. Relieve embarrassment of distal circulation in a circumferentially burned limb by escharotomy. Incision of the eschar to relieve edema pressure can be performed as an emergency procedure without anesthesia, because the incision is made in an insensitive full-thickness burn. The incision must extend across the entire length of the eschar in the lateral and/or medial line of the limb including the fingers and joints. The incision should be deep enough to allow the cut edges of the eschar to separate.

4. Circumferential burns of the thorax occasionally impair respiratory excusion. Bilateral, midaxillary escharotomy incisions should be considered if respiratory excursions are limited. Fasciotomy is seldom required. However, it may be necessary to restore circulation for patients with associated skeletal trauma, crush injury, high-voltage electrical injury, or burns involving tissue beneath the investing fascia.

G. Nasogastric Tube Insertion

Insert a nasogastric tube and attach it to suction if the patient experiences nausea, vomiting, or distention, or if burns involve more than 25% of the total body surface area.

H. Narcotics, Analgesics, and Sedatives

Narcotics, analgesics, and sedatives should be used **sparingly.** If narcotics are necessary, they should be administered in small, frequent doses by the intravenous route only. The severely burned patient may be restless and anxious from hypoxemia or hypovolemia rather than actual pain. Consequently, the patient will respond better to oxygen and increased fluid administration, respectively, rather than to narcotic analgesics or sedatives.

I. Wound Care

Partial-thickness (second-degree) burns are painful when air currents pass over the burned surface. Gently covering with clean linen will relieve the pain and deflect air currents. Do not break blisters or apply an antiseptic agent. Any applied medication must be removed before appropriate antibacterial topical agents can be applied. Application of cold compresses or ice may intensify shock. **Do not immerse or apply cold water to a patient with extensive burns.** If cold soaks are used, they should be applied for only 10 to 15 minutes for pain relief of second-degree burns of 10% or less of the body surface.

J. Antibiotics

Antibiotics are infrequently indicated in the early postburn period. Coexisting infections may require specific antibiotic therapy.

V. Special Burn Requirements

A. Chemical Burns

Reaction between tissue components and acids or alkalies release thermal energy, which is responsible for chemical burns. Chemicals that cause burns are usually acids or alkalis. The alkali burns are generally more serious than acid burns, because the alkalis penetrate more deeply. Removal of the chemical and immediate attention to wound care are essential.

Chemical burns are influenced by the duration of contact, concentration of the chemical, and amount of the agent. Irrigate with a neutral solution (water) immediately. Flush away the chemical with large amounts of water, using a shower or hose if available, for at least 20 to 30 minutes. Alkali burns require longer irrigation. If dry powder is still present on the skin, brush it away before irrigation with water. Neutralizing agents have no advantage over water lavage, because reaction with the neutralizing agent may itself produce heat and damage tissue further. Alkali burns to the eye require continuous irrigation during the first eight hours after the burn. A small-caliber cannula can be fixed in the palpebral sulcus for such irrigation.

B. Electrical Burns

Electrical burns result from a source of electrical power making contact with the patient's body. Electrical burns frequently are more serious than they appear on the surface. As the current passes through the body, muscles, nerves, and blood vessels may be destroyed while sparing skin because of its high resistance. Rhabdomyolysis results in myoglobin release, which can cause acute renal failure.

The immediate management of a patient with a significant electrical burn includes attention to the airway and breathing, establishment of an intravenous line, electrocardiographic monitoring, and placement of an indwelling urethral catheter. If the urine is dark, assume that myoglobin is present in the urine. Do not wait for laboratory confirmation before instituting therapy for myoglobinuria. Fluid administration should be increased to ensure a urinary output of at least 100 ml/hour. If the pigment does not clear with increased fluid administration, 25 gm of mannitol should be administered immediately and 12.5 gms of mannitol added to subsequent liters of fluid in order to maintain the diuresis.

Metabolic acidosis should be corrected by maintaining adequate perfusion and adding sodium bicarbonate in order to alkanize the urine and increase the solubility of myoglobin in the urine.

VI. Criteria for Transfer

A. Types of Burn Injuries

The American Burn Association has identified the following types of burn injuries that usually require referral to a burn center.

1. Partial-thickness and third-degree burns involving more than 10% of the total body surface area in patients under 10 years or over 50 years of age.

2. Partial-thickness and third-degree burns exceeding 20% of the body surface area in other age groups.

3. Partial-thickness and third-degree burns involving the face, eyes, ears, hands, feet, genitalia, perineum, and major joints.

4. Third-degree burns greater than 5% of the body surface area in any age group.

5. Electrical burns, including lightning injury. (Significant volumes of tissue beneath the surface may be injured and result in acute renal failure and other complications.)

6. Chemical burns.

7. Burns associated with significant fractures or other major injury in which the burn injury poses the greatest risk of morbidity or mortality.

8. Burn injury with inhalation injury.

9. Lesser burns in patients with significant pre-existing disease.

B. Transfer Procedure

1. Transfer of any patient must be coordinated with the burn-unit physician.

2. All pertinent information regarding tests, temperature, pulse, fluids administered, and urinary output should be recorded on the burn/trauma flow sheet and sent with the patient. Any other information deemed important by the referring or receiving physician is also sent with the patient.

VII. Cold Injury

Severity of cold injury depends on temperature, duration of exposure, and environmental conditions. Lower temperatures, immobilization, prolonged exposure, moisture, the presence of peripheral vascular disease, and open wounds all increase the severity of the injury.

A. Types

Three types of cold injury are seen in the trauma patient:

1. Frostbite, which is due to freezing of tissue from intracellular ice crystal formation and microvascular occlusion. Frostbite is classified, similarly to thermal burns, into first, second, third and fourth degree according to depth of involvement.

   a. First degree—Hyperemia, edema without skin necrosis.

   b. Second degree—Vesicle formation accompanies the hyperemia and edema with partial thickness necrosis of skin.

   c. Third degree—Full-thickness skin necrosis occurs, with necrosis of some underlying subcutaneous tissue.

   d. Fourth degree—Full-thickness skin necrosis including muscle and bone with gangrene.

2. **Nonfreezing** injury due to microvascular endothelial damage, stasis and vascular occlusion. With ambient temperature above freezing, prolonged exposure leads to "trench foot" over several days while "immersion foot" develops more slowly at higher temperatures. Although the entire foot may appear black, deep tissue destruction is not present. **Chilblain** or **pernio**, common among mountain climbers, results from exposure to dry temperatures just above freezing leading to superficial skin ulcers of the extremities.

3. **Hypothermia**—a state in which generalized core temperature depression below 35 degrees Centigrade occurs.

Depth of injury and extent of tissue damage is not usually accurate until demarcation is evident. This often requires several weeks of observation.

B. Management of Frostbite and Nonfreezing Cold Injuries

Treatment should be immediate to decrease duration of tissue freezing. Constricting, damp clothing should be replaced by warm blankets and the patient should be given hot fluids by mouth, if able to drink.

Place the injured part in circulating water at 40 degrees Centigrade until the pink color and perfusion return (usually within 20 to 30 minutes). Avoid dry heat.

C. Local Wound Care of Frostbite

The goal of wound care for frostbite is to preserve damaged tissue by preventing infection, avoiding opening noninfected vesicles, and elevating the injured area, which is left open to air. Narcotic analgesics are required.

Tetanus prophylaxis will depend on the patient's tetanus immunization status. Antibiotics are administered if infection is obviously present. Only rarely is fluid loss massive enough to require resuscitation with intravenous fluids.

VIII. Hypothermia

Total body hypothermia is defined as a core temperature below 35 degrees Centigrade. Clinically, hypothermia may be classified as mild (32 to 35 degrees Centigrade), moderate (30 to 32 degrees Centigrade), or severe (below 30 degrees).

This drop in core temperature may be rapid, as in immersion in near-freezing water; or slow, as in exposure to more temperate environments. The elderly are particularly susceptible to this condition, because of their impaired ability to increase heat production and decrease heat loss by vasoconstriction. Children are also more susceptible because of relative increased body surface area and limited energy sources. Since determination of the core temperature, preferably esophageal, is essential for the diagnosis, special thermometers capable of registering low temperatures are required.

A. Signs of Hypothermia

In addition to a decrease in core temperature, a depressed level of consciousness is the most common feature of hypothermia. The patient is cold to touch and appears gray and cyanotic. Vital signs, including pulse rate, respiratory rate, and blood pressure are all variable, and the absence of respiratory or cardiac activity is not uncommon in patients who eventually recover. Because of severe depression of the respiratory rate and heart rate, signs of respiratory and cardiac activity are easily missed unless careful assessment is conducted.

B. Management of Hypothermia

Immediate attention is paid to the ABCs, including the initiation of cardiopulmonary resuscitation and the establishment of intravenous access if the patient is in arrest. Intravenous access via peripheral veins may be difficult due to venous spasm, and may necessitate other access sites.

Prevent heat loss by removing the patient from the cold environment and replacing wet, cold clothing with warm blankets. Administer oxygen via a bag-reservoir device. The patient should be managed in a critical care setting whenever possible. A careful search for associated disorders, such as diabetes, sepsis, and drug or alcohol ingestion, should be conducted. These disorders should be treated promptly. Blood should be drawn for complete blood count, electrolytes, blood sugar, creatinine, amylase, and blood cultures. Abnormalities should be treated accordingly. For example, hypoglycemia would require intravenous glucose administration.

Determination of death can be very difficult in the hypothermic patient. While the patient's core temperature is still low, or for those patients who appear to be dead, pronouncement of death must be withheld until rewarming has been accomplished.

The rewarming technique depends on the patient's temperature and his response to simpler measures. For example, treat mild hypothermia (32 to 35 degrees Centigrade) by **passive external rewarming** in a warm room using warm blankets and clothing. Treat moderate hypothermia (30 to 32 degrees Centigrade) with warm intravenous fluids because of the patient's depressed level of consciousness. Loss of cardiac activity during rewarming or failure to elevate body temperature by 1 to 2 degrees Centigrade per hour requires **active core rewarming** methods, which may include invasive surgical rewarming techniques, eg, peritoneal lavage, thoracic/pleural lavage, hemodialysis, or cardiopulmonary bypass, all of which are better done in the critical care setting.

Cardiac drugs and defibrillation are not usually effective in the presence of acidosis, hypoxia, and hypothermia. Sodium bicarbonate and 100% oxygen should be administered while the patient is warmed to 32 degrees Centigrade, and cardiopulmonary resuscitation is continued. Cardiac drugs and defibrillation may then be instituted when the patient is rewarmed, as indicated.

Active external rewarming, including immersion in hot water (40 to 45 degrees Centigrade) and the use of electrical blankets, is controversial since it may lead to marked vasodilatation, hypotension, and cardiac dysrhythmias. This technique may be particularly dangerous in elderly patients.

IX. Summary

A. Burns–Thermal, Chemical, Electrical

Immediate life-saving measures for the burn patient include the **recognition of inhalation injury** and subsequent endotracheal intubation, and the rapid institution of intravenous fluid therapy. **All clothing should be removed rapidly.**

Early stabilization and management of the burn patient include:

1. Identifying the extent and depth of the burn.

2. Establishing fluid guidelines according to the patient's weight.

3. Initiating a patient-care flow sheet.

4. Obtaining baseline laboratory and roentgenographic studies.

5. Maintaining peripheral circulation in circumferential burns by performing an escharotomy if necessary.

6. Identifying which burn patients require transfer to a burn unit or center.

B. Cold Injuries

Diagnose the type of cold injury by obtaining an adequate history and noting the physical findings as well as measuring the core temperature using a low-range thermometer (esophageal temperature probe preferred). The patient should be removed from the cold environment immediately, and vital signs monitored and supported continuously. Rewarming techniques should be applied as soon as possible. For patients with hypothermia, the patient should not be considered dead until rewarming has occurred.

Figure 1

Depth of Burn	Signs & Symptoms	Severity
Second Degree Second-degree burns are deeper than first-degree burns, and involve partial thickness. They result from a very deep sunburn, contact with hot liquids, or flash burns from gasoline flames. They are usually more painful than third-degree burns. 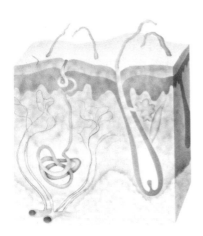	Red or mottled appearance. Blisters and broken epidermis. Considerable swelling. Weeping, wet surfaces. Painful. Sensitive to cold air.	**Critical:** Burns complicated by respiratory tract injury and fractures. Burns involving 15% to 30% of body surface. **Moderate:** Burns involving 15% to 30% of body surface. **Minor:** Burns of less than 15% of body surface.
Third Degree Third-degree burns cause damage to all skin layers, subcutaneous tissue, and nerve endings. They can be caused by fire, prolonged exposure to hot liquids, contact with hot objects or electricity. 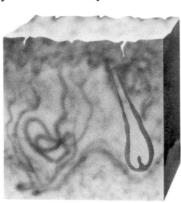	Pale white or charred apearance, leathery. (At first, may resemble second-degree burn.) Broken skin with fat exposed. Dry surface. Painless, insensitive to pinprick. Edema.	**Critical:** Burns complicated by respiratory tract injury and fractures. Burns involving the critical areas of the face, hands, or feet. Burns involving more than 10% of body surface. **Moderate:** Burns of 2% to 10% of body surface, and not involving face, hands, or feet. **Minor:** Burns of less than 2% of body surface.

Bibliography

1. Artz CP, Moncrief JA, Pruitt BA: **Burns, A Team Approach**. Philadelphia, WG Saunders, 1979.

2. Crapo RO: Smoke Inhalation Injuries. **Journal of the American Medical Association** 1981;246:1694.

3. Fein A, Leff A, Hopewell PC: Pathophysiology and Management of the Complications Resulting from Fire and the Inhaled Products of Combustion: Review of Literature. **Critical Care Medicine** 1980;8:94-98.

4. Guechot J, Lionet N, Cynober L, et al: Myoglobinemia After Burn Injury: Relationship to Creatine Kinase Activity in Serum. **Clinical Chemistry** 1986;32(5):857.

5. Munster AM: The Early Management of Thermal Burns. **Surgery** 1980;288:445-454.

6. Pruitt BA, Jr: The Burn Patient: I. Initial Care II. Late Care and Complications of Thermal Injury. **Current Problems in Surgery** April-May 1979;16:4&5

7. Reuler JB: Hypothermia: Pathophysiology, Clinical Settings and Management. **Annuals of Internal Medicine** 1978;89:519-27.

8. Sheehy TW, Navari RM: Hypothermia. **Intensive and Critical Care Digest** 1985;4:12-18.

Chapter 10:
Pediatric Trauma

Objectives:

Upon completion of this topic the participant will be able to:

A. Discuss the unique characteristics of the child as a trauma victim.

1. Types of injury
2. Patterns of injury
3. Long-term effects of injury

B. Discuss the pathophysiology of the following types of life-threatening situations.

1. Acute airway obstruction
2. Shock
3. Thoracic trauma
4. Abdominal trauma
5. Head and spinal trauma
6. Extremity trauma

C. Discuss the primary management of the following critical differences as directly related to the pediatric trauma victim.

1. Airway management
2. Fluid and electrolyte management
3. Nature and dosage of medications
4. Psychological support

D. Discuss the injury patterns associated with the battered/abused child.

E. Discuss and demonstrate in a simulated situation the following procedures for the pediatric trauma victim.

1. Endotracheal intubation
2. Intravenous access
3. Fluid and drug administration
4. Immobilization and management of extremity trauma

**Chapter 10:
Pediatric
Trauma**

I. Introduction

The multiply injured child has unique characteristics that are addressed in this chapter. The incidence of blunt versus penetrating trauma is highest in the pediatric population. Falls and vehicular accidents account for almost 80% of all pediatric injuries. Multisystem injury is the rule rather than the exception, and therefore all organ systems must be assumed to be injured until proven otherwise.

The unique anatomic characteristics of the pediatric population require special consideration in assessment and management of the pediatric trauma victim.

A. Size and Shape

The child's smaller size results in a "smaller target" to which are applied linear forces from fenders, bumpers and falls. The applied energy dissipates over the smaller mass of the child, resulting in greater force over a smaller area. This more intense energy is applied to a body with less body fat, less elastic connective tissue, and closer proximity of multiple organs, resulting in a high frequency of multiple organ injuries.

B. Skeleton

The child's skeleton is incompletely calcified, contains multiple active growth centers, and is more resilient. Therefore, it is less able to absorb significant forces applied during a traumatic event. This results in internal organ damage without overlying bony fracture. For example, rib fractures in the child are unusual, but pulmonary contusion is common.

C. Surface Area

The ratio between a child's body surface and body volume is highest at birth and diminishes throughout infancy and childhood. As a result, thermal energy loss becomes a significant stress factor in the smaller child. Hypothermia frequently adds additional stress to the hypotensive child, and may be life-threatening.

D. Psychological Status

Psychological ramifications of caring for an injured child can present significant challenges. In the very young child, emotional lability frequently leads to a regressive psychological behavior when stress, pain, or other perceived threats intervene in the child's environment. The child's ability to interact with unfamiliar individuals in strange environments is usually limited, making history-taking and cooperative manipulation extremely difficult. The physician who understands these characteristics and is willing to cajole and soothe an injured child is more likely to establish a good rapport, facilitating comprehensive assessment of the child's physiological state.

E. Long-Term Effects

A major consideration in dealing with injured children is the effect that injury may have on subsequent growth and development. Unlike the adult, the child must not only recover from the effects of a traumatic event, but must also continue the normal process of growth and development. The physiological and psychological effects of injury on this process should not be underestimated, particularly in those cases involving long-term function, growth deformity, or abnormal subsequent development. Children sustaining even a minor injury may have prolonged disability in either cerebral function, psychological adjustment, or organ system disability. Inadequate or inappropriate care in the immediate posttraumatic period may affect not only the child's survival, but perhaps just as importantly, the quality of the child's life for years to come.

F. Equipment

Immediately available equipment of the appropriate size is essential for successful initial management of the injured child. (See Table 4 at the end of this chapter.)

II. Airway Management

The primary goal of initial assessment and triage of the injured child is to restore adequate tissue oxygenation as effectively and completely as possible. Oxygenation and circulation are as essential to the injured child as to the adult. In this regard, the standard principles of airway control, breathing, and circulation are applied no differently to the injured child than to the injured adult. As always, the child's airway is the first priority of assessment.

A. Anatomy

The smaller the child, the greater the disproportion between size of cranium and midface, and the greater the propensity of the posterior pharyngeal area to "buckle," as the relatively larger occiput forces passive flexion of the cervical spine. As a result, the child's airway is best protected by a slightly superior anterior position of the midface, known as the "sniffing position." Careful attention to maintaining this position while affording maximum protection to the cervical spine is especially important in the obtunded child, whose level of consciousness is waxing and waning. In the infant, the tongue is relatively large compared to the oral cavity, which may make visualization of the larynx difficult.

A child's larynx is smaller than an adult's, has a slightly more antero-caudad angle, and is frequently more difficult to visualize for direct cannulation. The infant's trachea is short (5.0 cm) and grows to about 7.0 cm by about 18 months. Failure to appreciate this length may lead not only to bronchial intubation, but to hypoxia or perforation.

B. Management

In a spontaneously breathing child, the airway should be secured by the chin lift or jaw thrust maneuver. Supplemental oxygen should be delivered after the mouth and oropharynx have been cleared of secretions or debris. If the patient is unconscious, mechanical methods of maintaining the airway may be necessary.

1. Oral airway

The practice of inserting the airway backwards and rotating it 180 degrees is not recommended for the pediatric patient. Trauma to the teeth or soft-tissue structures of the oral pharynx may occur. Gently direct the oral airway into the oral pharynx, using a tongue blade to depress the tongue.

2. Orotracheal intubation

Endotracheal intubation is the most reliable means of ventilating the child with airway compromise. Uncuffed, specifically sized pediatric tubes should be used to avoid subglottic edema and ulceration. A simple technique to gauge the size of the endotracheal tube is to approximate the diameter of the child's external nares with the tube diameter. An alternate method is to equate the size of the child's fifth finger to the appropriate-sized tube for that child. Nasotracheal intubation requires blind passage around a relatively acute posterior nasopharyngeal angle and may cause inadvertent penetration of the cranial vault. For this reason, endotracheal intubation under direct vision with adequate immobilization and protection of the cervical spine is a more reliable means of obtaining initial airway control. Once passed, the endotracheal tube should be carefully positioned 2.0 to 3.0 cm below the level of the cords, and careful auscultation of both hemithoraces in the axillae should be done to assure adequate bilateral breath sounds. Breath sounds should be periodically rechecked, not only to ensure adequate positioning of the endotracheal tube, but also to rule out the possibility of evolving ventilatory dysfunction, secondary to excess tidal volume delivery to the tracheobronchial tree.

3. Cricothyroidotomy

Surgical cricothyroidotomy is rarely indicated for the infant or small child. When airway access and control cannot be accomplished by bag-valve-mask or oral endotracheal intubation, needle cricothyroidotomy is the preferred method. Needle jet insufflation via the cricothyroid membrane, as for adults, is an appropriate temporizing technique.

III. Shock

A. Recognition

Injury in childhood frequently results in significant blood loss. The increased physiologic reserve of the child may result in vital signs which are only slightly abnormal. The organs of primary importance in the child suffering hypovolemic shock are the heart, central nervous system, skin, and kidneys. Each can be monitored to identify the severity of the hypovolemia.

The primary response to hypovolemia in the child is tachycardia. Caution must be exercised when monitoring only heart rate, because tachycardia also can be caused by psychological stress, pain, and fear.

Hypovolemic shock in the pediatric patient can be described in terms of blood volume loss (normal blood volume = 80 ml/kg), and changes in monitored vital organ function (see Table 1).

Table 1

System Responses to Blood Loss
in the Pediatric Patient

	Early < 25% Blood Loss	Prehypotensive 25% Blood Volume Loss	Hypotensive 40% Blood Volume Loss
Cardiac	Weak, thready pulse, increased heart rate	+ Tilt test, increased heart rate	Frank hypotension, tachycardia to bradycardia
CNS	Lethargic, irritable, confused, combative	Changes in level of conciousness, dulled response to pain	Comatose
Skin	Cool, clammy	Cyanotic, decreased capillary refill, cold extremities	Pale, cold
Kidneys	Decreased urinary output ; increased specific	Increased BUN	No urinary output

Although signs of frank hypovolemic shock may be unmistakable, minimal or evolving shock may be extremely subtle, demanding careful observation. The association of tachycardia, cool extremities, and a systolic blood pressure of less than 70 mmHg are clear indications of evolving shock. A child's systolic blood pressure should be 80 plus twice the age in years, and diastolic pressure two-thirds of the systolic blood pressure.

Vital signs for the child are age-related. Hence knowledge of normal vital signs is important (see Table 2).

Table 2

Vital Signs

	P (rate/ minute)	BP (mmHg)	R (rate/ minute)
Infant	160	80	40
Preschool	140	90	30
Adolescent	120	100	20

B. Fluid Resuscitation

Fluid resuscitation for the child follows the same basic principles as for the adult. Because approximately 25% of blood volume diminution is required to begin manifestations of shock, a fluid challenge of 20 ml/kg, which represents 25% of the normal blood volume of a child (80 ml/kg or 8% of body weight) is an appropriate initial bolus. The same "three-for-one" rule used to estimate crystalloid replacement for the adult patient also applies to the pediatric patient. To achieve a 25% blood volume replacement in the child requires 60 ml/kg of crystalloid fluid. Routine fluid maintenance for the injured child is outside the first hour of care. The resuscitation flow diagram is a useful aid for the initial management of the injured child. (See Table 3.)

Failure to obtain hemodynamic stability following the first bolus of resuscitation fluid mandates prompt involvement of the surgeon, if such an individual is not already involved.

Table 3
Resuscitation Flow Diagram
for the Stable and Unstable Pediatric Patient

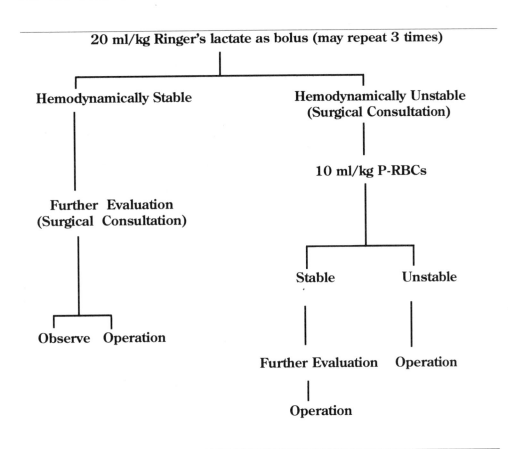

C. Blood Replacement

The child in severe hypovolemic shock who responds to an initial crystalloid bolus must have restitution of this circulating red cell volume to ensure adequate tissue oxygenation. Rapid red cell transfusion of preferably warm, fresh blood should be considered as soon as adequate venous access has been established, and the patient has been determined to be severely hypovolemic. Children who have received two trial boluses of 20 ml/kg of Ringer's lactate and have not responded, clearly require ongoing crystalloid and immediate blood transfusion. Until type-specific blood is available, type-O, Rh-negative packed red cells (10 ml/kg) or type-specific whole blood (20 ml/kg) should be transfused.

Note: Blood transfusion is not without inherent risks. It is strongly recommended that if a child with a suspected injured spleen or liver requires 10 ml/kg of blood for stabilization, expeditious celiotomy should be undertaken to avoid the added risks of blood transfusion. (See Table 3.)

D. Acid-Base Complications

In pediatric resuscitation, the most common acid-base abnormality develops secondarily to hypoventilation. Children for whom adequate ventilation and perfusion are established should be able to maintain a relatively normal pH. However, should the pH fall below 7.2, sodium bicarbonate may need to be added to the fluid replacement. The formula for calculating the dose of sodium bicarbonate is:

Body weight in kg (0.3) (base deficit) = Total $NaHCO_3$ dose

One half of this may be given as an intravenous bolus and the rest administered at a rate of three to five mEq/minute after adequate ventilation has been established. In the absence of adequate ventilation, $NaHCO_3$ will **not** correct the evolving acidosis.

E. Venous Access

Severe hypovolemic shock usually occurs as a result of disruption of intrathoracic or intra-abdominal organ systems. Venous access should be established initially via a percutaneous route if possible. If this route is unsuccessful, a direct cutdown should be considered at the the following sites:

1. Greater saphenous at the ankle
2. Median cephalic at the elbow
3. Main cephalic higher in the upper arm
4. External jugular
5. Long bone marrow (intraosseous infusion)

Intravenous access in the hypovolemic child under six years of age is a perplexing and difficult problem, even in the most experienced hands. **Intraosseous infusion,** cannulating the marrow cavity of a long bone in an uninjured extremity, is an emergency "intravenous" access procedure for the critically ill and injured pediatric patient. The intraosseous route is safe, efficacious, and requires less time than venous cutdown. Indications for this procedure include the child, six years of age or younger, for whom venous access is impossible due to circulatory collapse; or vein cannulation has failed on two attempts. Complications of this procedure include cellulitis and very rarely, osteomyelitis.

The preferred site for intraosseous cannulation is the anterior tibial plateau, 2 to 3 cm below the tibial tuberosity. If the tibia is fractured, the intravenous catheter may be inserted into the inferior third of the femur, 3 cm above the external condyle, anterior to the midline. Intraosseous cannulation should not be done distal to a fracture site.

Using a #16- to #18-gauge (one-half inch in length) bone marrow aspiration/transfusion needle, entry is perpendicular to the bone or 60 degrees inferiorly with the bevel directed up. Aspiration of bone marrow identifies adequate needle position. Crystalloids, blood products, and drugs (except Bretylium) can be administered via the intraosseous route. Circulation time from marrow cavity to the heart is generally less than 20 seconds. Volume resuscitation can be accomplished in an acceptable period of time by this method.

F. Thermoregulation

The high ratio of body surface to body mass in children increases the facility with which heat exchange occurs, and directly affects their ability to regulate core temperature. Thin skin and the lack of substantial subcutaneous tissue contribute to increased evaporative heat loss and calorie expenditure. The small patient who is hypothermic may be refractory to therapy for shock. While the child is exposed during the initial survey and resuscitation phase, overhead heaters or thermal blankets may be necessary to maintain body temperature.

IV. Chest Trauma

Adults frequently sustain penetrating and blunt chest injuries. However, in the preadolescent child, penetrating thoracic injury is rare. Blunt thoracic trauma is common in children and often requires immediate correction of function to establish adequate ventilation. The child's chest wall, which is very compliant, allows energy to transfer to the intrathoracic structures, frequently without any evidence of injury on the external chest wall. The specific problems caused by thoracic trauma in the child are not any different from those encountered in the adult, and usually can be treated without thoracotomy.

Tension pneumothorax or hemopneumothorax, the result of high-energy accidents, are **not** well-tolerated by the child due to the mobility of the mediastinal structures. This mobility also makes the child especially sensitive to **flail segments.** The elastic chest wall increases the frequency of pulmonary contusions and direct intrapulmonary hemorrhage, usually without overlying rib fractures.

Children sustain bronchial injuries and diaphragmatic ruptures with some frequency due to blunt, crushing forces. **Injury to the great vessels** is infrequent compared to the adult experience, which may reflect a lack of organic vascular disease.

The diagnostic and therapeutic approach to chest trauma is the same for children and adults. Significant thoracic injuries rarely occur alone and are often a component of major multisystem injury.

V. Abdominal Trauma

As with chest injuries, most pediatric abdominal injuries are associated with blunt trauma.

A. Assessment

The conscious infant and young child obviously will be greatly frightened by the events preceding admission to the emergency department. While talking quietly and calmly to the child, ask questions about the presence of abdominal pain, and gently assess the tone of the abdominal musculature. Avoid deep palpation at the onset of the examination where the pain is centered, as the child will voluntarily guard against subsequent abdominal compression. Almost all infants and young children who are stressed and crying will swallow a large amount of air. Prior to any further evaluation, decompress the stomach by inserting a gastric tube. Tenseness of the abdominal wall will often decrease as gastric distention is relieved. The abdomen should then be reevaluated. Abdominal examination in the unconscious patient will not vary greatly with age. The insertion of gastric and urinary catheters will simplify the examination.

B. Peritoneal Lavage

The indications for peritoneal lavage and the interpretation of results are the same for pediatric and adult patients, but peritoneal lavage is needed less often for children.

Remember, use a buffered Ringer's lactate solution in the dosage of 10 ml/kg up to 1,000 ml, with the solution running over a 10-minute period. **Note:** The child's abdominal wall is much thinner than the adult's. Sudden penetration of the abdominal wall can be dangerous, even using the open technique.

C. Computed Tomography Scan

Many pediatric trauma centers use computed tomographic (CT) scanning in place of peritoneal lavage. Some use the CT scan with the diagnostic peritoneal lavage. If the CT scan is used for pediatric blunt abdominal trauma, it must be immediately available and not delay further treatment.

D. Nonoperative Management

Some trauma centers are evaluating nonoperative management of children with blunt trauma. They must be managed in a facility offering pediatric intensive-care capabilities, and under the supervision of a qualified pediatric surgeon. Intensive care must include continuous nursing staff coverage, monitoring of vital signs either continuously or every 15 minutes, and **immediate** availability of surgical personnel and operating room facilities. When celiotomy is required, injuries to the spleen and liver in children can frequently be repaired **without** sacrificing the spleen or resecting lobes of the liver.

VI. Head Trauma

Information provided in Chapter 6–Head Trauma, also applies to pediatric patients. This chapter emphasizes additional points peculiar to children.

A. Assessment

Children and adults may differ in their response to head trauma, affecting evaluation of an injured child. The principal differences are:

1. Although children generally recover better than adults, children less than three years old have worse outcomes from severe head injury than older children. **Secondary brain injury from hypoxemia and hypovolemia must be avoided.**

2. Although an infrequent occurrence, **infants may become hypotensive from a head injury due to blood loss** into either the subgaleal or epidural space. Always consider hypovolemia and provide appropriate volume resuscitation.

3. The young child with an open fontanelle and mobile sutures is more tolerant of an expanding intracranial mass. Other signs of an expanding mass may be hidden until rapid decompensation occurs. Therefore, a bulging fontanelle or sutural diastasis in an infant who is not in coma should be treated as a more severe injury.

4. Vomiting is common after head injury in children, and does not necessarily mean increased intracranial pressure. However, persistent vomiting or vomiting that worsens is of concern, and demands computed tomography scanning.

5. Seizures occurring shortly after injury are more common in children. They usually are self-limiting. Recurring seizures require investigation by computed tomography scanning.

6. Children tend to have fewer focal mass lesions than adults. But elevated intracranial pressure without masses is more common. In children, a lucid interval or delayed neurological deterioration occurs more commonly from brain swelling and high, increased intracranial pressure. Therefore, emergency computed tomography scanning is vital to diagnose those children who require emergency surgery.

7. The Glasgow Coma Scale score is useful when applied to the pediatric age group. However, the verbal score must be modified, as follows, for very young children.

Verbal Response	V-Score
Appropriate words or social smile, fixes and follows.	5
Cries, but consolable	4
Persistently irritable	3
Restless, agitated	2
None	1

8. Because of the frequency for increased intracranial pressure in children, intracranial pressure monitoring is frequently undertaken very early in resuscitation. Some indications are:

  a. Children with a Glasgow Coma Scale of five or less, or motor scores of one or two.

  b. Multiply injured children who require major volume resuscitation, immediate life-saving thoracic or abdominal surgery, or for whom stabilization or assessment will be prolonged and computed tomography scan will be delayed.

9. The following medication doses must be given as dictated by the size of the child.

  a. Diazepam–0.25 mg/kg, IV slow push.

  b. Phenytoin–15 to 20 mg/kg, administered at 0.5 to 1.5 mg/kg/minute loading, then 4 to 7 mg/kg/day maintenance.

  c. Mannitol–0.5 to 1.0gm/kg.

B. Management

Successful management of pediatric brain injury involves:

1. Using appropriate pediatric specialists from the beginning of treatment.

2. Rapid, early assessment and management of the airway and circulatory systems.

3. Appropriate, sequential assessment and management of the brain injury to prevent secondary injuries, ie, hypoxia and ischemia. Early endotracheal intubation with adequate oxygenation and ventilation is indicated to avoid further central nervous system damage due to secondary brain injury.

4. Continuous reassessment of all parameters.

VII. Spinal Cord Injury

Information provided in Chapter 7–Spine and Spinal Cord Trauma, also applies to pediatric patients. This chapter emphasizes the peculiarities of pediatric spinal injury.

Pediatric spinal cord injury is rare. Only 5% of all spinal cord injuries occur in the pediatric age group. For children less than ten years of age, motor vehicle accidents most commonly cause spinal cord injury. For children ages 10 to 14 years, motor vehicle accidents and sporting accidents, both recreational and organized, account for an equal number of spinal injuries.

A. Anatomical Differences

1. Interspinous ligaments and joint capsules are more flexible.

2. The uncinate articulations are poorly developed and incompetent.

3. Vertebral bodies are wedged anteriorly, and tend to slide forward with flexion.

4. The facet joints are flat.

5. The child has a relatively large head compared to the adult, and more angular momentum can be generated during flexion or extension.

B. Radiographic Considerations

Pseudosubluxation—About 40% of young children (ie, less than seven years of age) show anterior displacement of C-2 on C-3. About 20% of children up to age sixteen exhibit this phenomenon. This injury is seen less commonly at C-3-4. More than 3 mm of movement is exhibited at these joints when they are studies by flexion and extension maneuvers.

Increased distance between the dens and anterior arch of C-1 occurs in about 20% of young children. Gaps exceeding the upper limit for the adult age group are frequently seen.

Skeletal growth centers can resemble fractures. Basilar odontoid synchrondrosis appears as a radiolucent line at the base of the dens, especially in children less than five years of age. Apical odontoid epiphyses appear as separations on the odontoid roentgenogram, and are seen usually between the ages of 5 to 11. The growth center of the spinous processes rarely may resemble fractures of the tip of the spinous process.

More commonly than adults, children can suffer spinal cord injury with no radiographic abnormality. A normal spine film or spine series can be found in up to two thirds of children suffering spinal cord injury. When spinal cord injury is suspected, based on the neurologic examination or history, the findings of plain radiographic studies should not deter the physician's diagnosis.

VIII. Extremity Trauma

The initial priorities in the management of skeletal trauma in the child are similar to those for the adult, with the addition of concerns about potential injury to the growth plate.

A. History

History is of vital importance. In the younger child, roentgenographic diagnosis of fractures and dislocations around the joint are difficult because of the lack of mineralization of the epiphysis and presence of a physis (growth plate). Occasionally roentgenograms of the opposite extremity may be useful for comparison.

Information about the magnitude, mechanism, and time of the injury facilitates better correlation of the physical findings and roentgenograms. Old, healed fractures should alert the physician to possible child abuse.

B. Blood Loss

Blood loss associated with long-bone and pelvic fractures is proportionately greater in the child than in the adult. Even a small child can lose up to one unit of blood into the muscle mass or thigh and develop hemodynamic instability as the result of a fractured femur.

C. Physeal (Growth Plate) Fractures

Bone grows in length as new bone is laid down by the growth plate or physis near the end of the bone. The area immediately adjacent to the physis is called the metaphysis; the middle of a long bone is called the diaphysis. The area of the bone distal to the physis is called the epiphysis. For a child whose growth plate is not closed, there is a potential for further bone growth. An injury near a joint will lead to a fracture through the physis. Physeal fractures have been classified by the Salter-Harris method as types I through V. The potential for growth disturbances is increased with the progressive types.

1. Physeal fractures that shear transversely through the growth plate and those that carry a small chip of metaphysis have the best prognosis for continued normal growth (types I and II).

2. Fractures that pass obliquely through the epiphysis (type III) or through both epiphysis and the metaphysis (type IV) have a relatively higher incidence of subsequent growth deformity.

3. Compression fractures (type V), which may be difficult to recognize on roentgenograms, severely compress the physis and have the worst prognosis for subsequent normal growth.

D. "Greenstick" Fracture

Because of the nature of immature bones, only one cortex of the long bone may fracture. This is called a "greenstick" fracture. In these cases, the bone usually must be fractured entirely through both cortices before casting.

E. Buckle Fracture

A torus or "buckle" fracture is seen exclusively in small children. It is an angulation deformity of the relatively malleable bones of a young child without actual fracture of the bone. Mild angulation is acceptable in a child.

F. Supracondylar Fracture

Supracondylar fractures at the elbow have a high propensity for vascular injury and an increased incidence of growth deformity. They may be confused with dislocations at the elbow. Fractures of the lateral condyle of the distal humerus also have a propensity for growth deformity.

IX. The Battered, Abused Child

The battered child syndrome or physical child abuse refers to any child who sustains a nonaccidental injury as the result of acts by parents, guardians, or acquaintances. Most children who die of abuse have had multiple, recurring episodes of battering. Therefore, a history and careful evaluation of the child suspected of being abused, is critically important to prevent eventual death. A physician should suspect abuse if:

1. A discrepancy exists between the history and the degree of physical injury.

2. A prolonged interval has passed between the time of the injury and the seeking of medical advice.

3. The history includes repeated trauma, treated in different emergency rooms.

4. Parents respond inappropriately to or do not comply with medical advice, eg, leaving a child in the emergency facility.

5. The history of injury changes or differs between parents or guardians.

These findings, on careful physical examination, should suggest child abuse and indicate more intensive investigation:

1. Multiple subdural hematomas, especially without a fresh skull fracture.

2. Retinal hemorrhage.

3. Perioral injuries.

4. Ruptured internal viscera without antecedent major blunt trauma.

5. Trauma to the genital or perianal areas.

6. Evidence of frequent injuries typified by old scars or healed fractures on roentgenogram.

7. Fractures of long bones in children under three years of age.

8. Bizarre injuries such as bites, cigarette burns, or rope marks.

9. Sharply demarcated second- and third-degree burns in unusual areas.

The physician's primary responsibility is to treat and aggressively resuscitate the battered child, but the next priority is to bring any suspicious situation to the attention of appropriate personnel and child-abuse teams. The physician bears the legal responsibility for identifying such patients and notifying proper authorities, so that an appropriate investigation can be carried out and the child protected from further abuse.

X. Summary

The recognition and management of pediatric injuries requires the same astute skills as for adults. However, the unwary physician can make grievous errors unless he is fully cognizant of the unique features of the pediatric trauma patient. These unique characteristics include airway anatomy and management; fluid requirements; diagnosis of exclusive extremity fractures; and the recognition of the battered, abused child.

Table 4
Pediatric Equipment

Age Weight (kg)	Airway/Breathing							Circulation		Supplemental Equipment			
	O₂ Mask	Oral Airways	Bag-Valve Mask	Laryngo-scope Blades	ET Tubes	Stylet	Suction	BP Cuff	IV Catheter	NG Tubes	Chest Tubes	Foleys Urine Collector	C-collar
Premie 3 kg	Premie Newborn	Infant	Infant	0 — Straight	2.5-3.0 Uncuffed	6 Fr	6-8 Fr	Premie Newborn	22 Gauge	12 Fr Anderson	10-14 Fr	5 Fr Feeding	—
Newborn 0-6 mos 3.5 kg	NB	Infant Small	Infant	1 — Straight	3.0-3.5 Uncuffed	6 Fr	8 Fr	Newborn Infant	22 Gauge	12 Fr Anderson	12-18 Fr	5-8 Fr Feeding	—
6-12 mos 7 kg	PED	Small	PED	1 — Straight	3.5-4.5 Uncuffed	6 Fr	8-10 Fr	Infant Child	22 Gauge	12 Fr Anderson	14-20 Fr	8 Fr	Small
1-3 yrs. 10-12 kg	PED	Small	PED	1 — Straight	4.0-4.5 Uncuffed	6 Fr	10 Fr	Child	20-22 Gauge	12 Fr Anderson	14-24 Fr	10 Fr	Small
4-7 yrs. 16-18 kg	PED	Medium	PED	2 — Straight or Curved	5.0-5.5 Uncuffed	14 Fr	14 Fr	Child	20 Gauge	12 Fr Anderson	20-32 Fr	10-12 Fr	Small
8-10 yrs. 24-30 kg	Adult	Medium Large	PED Adult	2-3 — Straight or Curved	5.5-6.5 Cuffed	14 Fr	14 Fr	Child Adult	18-20 Gauge	12 Fr Anderson	28-38 Fr	12 Fr	Medium

Bibliography

1. Becker D, et al: The Outcome From Severe Head Injury with Early Diagnosis and Intensive Management. **Journal of Neurosurgery** 1977;47:491.

2. Bruce D: Outcome Following Severe Head Injuries in Children. **Journal of Neurosurgery** 1978;48:697.

3. Bruce DA, Raphaely RC, Goldberg AI, et al: Pathophysiology, Treatment and Outcome Following Severe Head Injury in Children. **Child's Brain**1979;5:174-191.

4. Cattell HS, Filter DL: Pseudosubluxation and Other Normal Variations in the Cervical Spine in Children. **Journal Bone and Joint Surgery (AM)** 1965;47:1296-1309.

5. Chesire DJE: The Paediatric Syndrome of Traumatic Myelopathy without Demonstrable Vertebral Injury. **Paraplegia** 1977;15:74-85.

6. Gross CR, Wolf C, Kunitz SC, et al: Pilot Traumatic Coma Data Bank: A Profile of Head Injuries in Children, in Dacy RG, Winn HR, Rimel RW, Jane JA (eds)**Journal of the Central Nervous System**. New York, Raven Press, 1985, pp 19-26.

7. Hill SA, Miller CA, Kosnik EJ, et al: Pediatric Neck Injuries. **Journal of Neurosurgery** 1984;60:700-706.

8. Kewalramani LS, Tori JA: Spinal Cord Trauma in Children.**Spine** 1980;5:11-18.

9. Kraus JF, Fife D, Cox P, et al: Incidence, Severity and External Causes of Pediatric Brain Injury. **AJDC** 1986;140:687-693.

10. Luerssen TG: Resuscitation of Brain-Injured Children: Special Considerations. **Trauma Quarterly** 1985;2:20-25.

11. Luna GK, Dellinger EP: Nonoperative Observation Therapy for Splenic Injuries: A Safe Therapeutic Option. **American Journal of Surgery** 1987;153:462-468.

12. O'Neill JA, Meacham WF, Griffin PO, et al: Patterns of Injury in the Battered Children Syndrome. **Journal of Trauma** 1973;13:332.

13. Pang D, Wilberger JE: Spinal Cord Injury without Radiographic Abnormalities in Children. **Journal of Neurosurgery** 1982;57:114-129.

14. Powell RW, Green JB, et al: Peritoneal Lavage in Pediatric Patients Sustaining Blunt Abdominal Trauma: A Reappraisal. **Journal of Trauma** 1987;27:1.

15. Ramenofsky ML, Luterman A, et al: Maximum Survival in Pediatric Trauma: The Ideal System. **Journal of Trauma** 1984;24(9):818.

16. Shires GT, Canizaro PC: Fluid Resuscitation in the Severely Injured Child. **Surgical Clinics of North America** 1973;53:1341.

17. Tepas JJ, Ramenofsky ML, et al: The Pediatric Trauma Score as a Prediction of Injury Severity: An Objective Assessment. **Journal of Trauma,** 1987 (In press).

18. Walker ML, Mayer TA, Storrs BB et al: Pediatric Head Injury–Factors which Influence Outcome, in Chapman, PH (ed). **Concepts in Pediatric Neurosurgery VI** Basel:Karger, 1985, pp 84-97.

Chapter 11:
Trauma in Pregnancy

Objectives:

Upon completion of this topic the participant will be able to discuss the primary management of the following critical aspects of the care of the pregnant trauma patient.

A. Oxygen requirements

B. Blood replacement requirements

C. Proper patient positioning

D. Significance of fetal monitoring

E. Vaginal bleeding

**Chapter 11:
Trauma in
Pregnancy**

I. Introduction

Pregnancy causes major physiologic changes and altered anatomic relationships involving nearly every organ system of the body. These changes of structure and function may influence the evaluation of the traumatized pregnant patient by altering the signs and symptoms of injury, as well as the results of diagnostic laboratory tests. Pregnancy may also affect the patterns of injury or severity of injury. **Treatment priorities for an injured pregnant patient remain the same as for the nonpregnant patient.** The best treatment for the fetus is to treat the mother. However, resuscitation and stabilization should be modified to accommodate the unique anatomic and physiologic changes of pregnancy. The physician attending a pregnant trauma victim must remember that he does, in fact, have two patients. A thorough understanding of this special relationship between a pregnant patient and her fetus is essential if the best interests of both are to be served. The use of roentgenograms, if indicated during critical management, should not be withheld because of the pregnancy. A qualified obstetrician should be consulted early in the evaluation of the pregnant trauma victim.

II. Anatomic and Physiologic Alterations of Pregnancy

A. Anatomic

The uterus remains an intrapelvic organ until the twelfth week of gestation, when it begins to rise out of the pelvis and encroach on the peritoneal cavity. By 20 weeks, the uterus is at the umbilicus. At 36 weeks, it reaches its maximal supraumbilical extent—the costal margin. During the last two to eight weeks of gestation, the fetus slowly descends as the fetal head engages the pelvis. As the uterus enlarges, it reduces the confines of the intraperitoneal space, restricting the intestines to the upper abdomen. Likewise, the intrauterine environment gradually changes from very protective to very vulnerable. During the first trimester, the uterus is a thick-walled structure of limited size, confined within the safety of the bony pelvis. During the second trimester, the uterus leaves its protected intrapelvic location, but the small fetus remains mobile and cushioned by a relatively generous amount of amniotic fluid. By the third trimester, the uterus is large and thin-walled. The head is usually fixed in the pelvis with the remainder of the fetus exposed above the pelvic brim. The placenta reaches its maximum size by 36 to 38 weeks, and is devoid of elastic tissue. The placental vasculature is maximally dilated throughout gestation, yet is exquisitely sensitive to catecholamine stimulation. Direct trauma to the placenta or uterus may reverse the normal protective hemostasis of pregnancy by releasing high concentrations of placental thromboplastin or plasminogen activator from the myometrium. All of these changes make the uterus and its contents more susceptible to injury, including penetration, rupture, abruptio placenta, and premature rupture of membranes.

B. Hemodynamic

1. Cardiac output

After the tenth week of pregnancy, cardiac output is increased by 1.0 to 1.5 liters per minute. This increased output is greatly influenced by the maternal position as term nears. Vena cava compression in the supine position may decrease cardiac output by 30% to 40%.

2. Heart rate

Heart rate increases throughout pregnancy. During the third trimester, it reaches a rate of 15 to 20 beats per minute more than in the nonpregnant state.

3. Blood pressure

Pregnancy results in a 5- to 15-mmHg fall in systolic and diastolic pressures during the second trimester. Blood pressure returns to near-normal levels at term. Some women may exhibit profound hypotension (supine hypotensive syndrome) when placed in the supine position. This condition is relieved by turning the patient to the left lateral decubitus position.

4. Venous pressure

The resting CVP is variable with pregnancy, but the response to volume is the same as in the nonpregnant state. Venous hypertension in the lower extremities is normal during the third trimester.

5. Electrocardiographic changes

The axis may shift leftward by approximately 15 degrees. Flattened or inverted T-waves in leads III, AVF and the precordial leads may be normal. Ectopic beats are increased during pregnancy.

C. Blood Volume and Composition

1. Volume

At 34 weeks gestation, plasma volume reaches a level of 40% to 50% more than prepregnancy. A smaller increase in RBC volume occurs, resulting in a decreased hematocrit (physiologic anemia of pregnancy). In late pregnancy, a hematocrit of 31% to 35% is normal. Blood volume overall increases by 48%. With hemorrhage, otherwise healthy pregnant women may lose 30% to 35% of their blood volume before exhibiting symptoms.

2. Composition

The WBC count increases during pregnancy to a high of 20,000. Serum fibrinogen and many clotting factors are elevated. Prothrombin and partial thromboplastin times may be shortened, but bleeding and clotting times are unchanged. Serum albumin falls to 2.2 to 2.8 g/dl during pregnancy, causing a drop in serum protein levels by approximately 1.0 g/dl. Serum osmolarity remains at about 280 mOsm/L throughout pregnancy.

D. Respiratory

The respiratory rate is not altered by pregnancy. Tidal volume increases by 40%, and the residual volume falls. This "hyperventilation" of pregnancy yields a PCO_2 of 30 mmHg late in gestation. During pregnancy, the chest roentgenogram shows increased lung markings from diaphragmatic elevation and increased prominence of pulmonary vessels.

E. Gastrointestinal

Gastric emptying is greatly prolonged during pregnancy, and the physician should assume that the stomach is full. The intestines are relocated to the upper abdomen and may be shielded by the uterus. The spleen and liver are essentially unchanged by pregnancy.

F. Urinary

The glomerular filtration rate and the renal plasma blood flow increase during pregnancy. Levels of creatinine and BUN fall to approximately one half of normal prepregnancy levels. Glycosuria is common during pregnancy. Excretory urography reveals a physiologic dilatation of the renal calyxes, pelves, and ureters outside of the pelvis.

G. Endocrine

The pituitary gland gets 30% to 50% heavier during pregnancy. Shock may cause necrosis of the anterior pituitary, resulting in pituitary insufficiency (Sheehan's syndrome).

H. Musculoskeletal

The symphysis pubis widens by the seventh month (4 to 8 mm). The sacral iliac joints also relax.

I. Neurologic

Eclampsia is a complication of late pregnancy that may mimic head injury. Eclampsia should be considered if seizures occur with or without hypertension, especially if hyperreflexia is present.

III. Diagnosis and Management

A. Initial Assessment

1. Patient position

Uterine compression of the vena cava reduces venous return to the heart, thereby decreasing cardiac output and aggravating the shock state. Elevated caval pressures below the point of compression can lead to extension of placental separation. Therefore, unless a spinal injury is suspected, the pregnant patient should be transported and evaluated on her left side. If the patient is supine, the right hip should be elevated and the uterus manually displaced to the left side, to relieve pressure on the inferior vena cava.

2. Primary survey

Follow the ABCs. Supplemental oxygen is administered. If ventilatory support is required, consideration should be given to hyperventilating the patient. Because of the increased intravascular volume and the rapid contraction of the uteroplacental circulation shunting blood away from the fetus, the pregnant patient can lose up to 35% of her blood volume before tachycardia, hypotension, and other signs of hypovolemia occur. Thus, the fetus may be "in shock" and deprived of vital perfusion, while the mother's condition and vital signs appear stable. Crystalloid fluid resuscitation and early type-specific blood administration is indicated to support the physiologic hypervolemia of pregnancy. Avoid administering vasopressors to restore maternal blood pressure, because these agents further reduce uterine blood flow, resulting in fetal hypoxia.

B. Secondary Assessment

The examination of the patient should include an assessment of uterine irritability, fundal height and tenderness, fetal heart tones, and fetal movement. Use a Doppler ultrasound stethoscope or fetoscope to auscultate fetal heart tones. Pay careful attention to the presence of uterine contractions, suggesting early labor; or tetanic contractions accompanied by vaginal bleeding, suggesting premature separation of the normally implanted placenta. The evaluation of the perineum should include a formal pelvic examination. The presence of amniotic fluid in the vagina, evidenced by a pH of 7 to 7.5, suggests ruptured chorio-amniotic membranes. Cervical effacement and dilatation, fetal presentation, and the relationship of the fetal presenting part to the ischial spines should be noted. Because vaginal bleeding in the third trimester may indicate disruption of the placenta and impending death of the fetus, an obstetrician ideally should carry out the vaginal examination, or be called immediately if blood is coming from the cervical os. The decision regarding an emergency cesarean section should be made in conjunction with an obstetrician.

C. Monitoring

1. Patient

If possible, the patient should be monitored on her left side after physical examination. Monitoring of the central venous pressure response to fluid challenge is extremely valuable in maintaining the relative hypervolemia required in pregnancy.

2. Fetus

Fetal distress can occur any time and without warning. Although fetal heart rate can be determined with any stethoscope, the fetal heart rate and rhythm is best monitored continuously using the ultrasonic Doppler cardioscope. The fetus should be continually monitored to ensure early recognition of fetal distress. Inadequate accelerations of fetal heart rate in response to fetal movement or late decelerations of fetal heart rate in response to uterine contractions indicate fetal hypoxia.

Indicated radiographic studies should be performed, because the benefits certainly outweigh potential risk to the fetus. However, unnecessary duplication of films should be avoided.

D. Definitive Care

In addition to the spectrum of injury found in a nonpregnant patient, trauma during pregnancy may cause uterine rupture. The uterus is protected by the bony pelvis in the first trimester, but becomes increasingly susceptible to injury as gestation progresses. Traumatic rupture may present a varied clinical picture. Massive hemorrhage and shock may be present, or only fairly minimal signs and symptoms may be present.

Radiographic evidence of rupture includes extended fetal extremities, abnormal fetal position, or free intraperitoneal air. Suspicion of uterine rupture mandates surgical exploration. Placental separation from the uterine wall (abruptio placenta) is the leading cause of fetal death after blunt trauma. With separation involving 25% of the placental surface, external vaginal bleeding and premature labor may begin. Larger areas of placental detachment are associated with increasing fetal distress and demise. Other than external bleeding, signs and symptoms may include abdominal pain, uterine tenderness, uterine rigidity, expanding fundal height, and maternal shock.

With extensive placental separation, or with amniotic fluid embolization, widespread intravascular clotting may develop, causing depletion of fibrinogen, other clotting factors, and platelets. This consumptive coagulopathy may emerge rapidly.

The large, engorged pelvic vessels that surround the gravid uterus can contribute to massive retroperitoneal bleeding after blunt trauma with associated pelvic fractures.

Initial management is directed at resuscitation and stabilization of the pregnant patient, because the fetus' life at this point is totally dependent on the integrity of the mother's. Fetal monitoring should be maintained after satisfactory resuscitation and stabilization of the mother.

Obstetrical consultation is in order, to aid in the definitive care of the fetus.

IV. Summary

Important and predictable anatomic and physiologic changes occur during pregnancy, which may influence the evaluation and treatment of the traumatized pregnant patient. Vigorous fluid and blood replacement should be given to correct and prevent maternal as well as fetal hypovolemic shock. A search should be made for conditions unique to the injured pregnant patient, such as blunt or penetrating uterine trauma, abruptio placenta, and premature rupture of membranes. Attention must also be directed toward the second patient of this unique duo–the fetus–after its environment has been stabilized. A qualified surgeon/obstetrician should be consulted early in the evaluation of the pregnant trauma patient.

Bibliography

1. Buchsbaum HJ: **Trauma in Pregnancy**. Philadelphia, WB Saunders Co, 1979.

2. Maull KI, Rozycki GS, Pedigo RE, et al: Female reproductive system trauma, in Moore EE, Feliciano DV, Mattox KL (eds): **Trauma**. Norwalk CT, Appleton-Lange,1987, pp 553-560.

Chapter 12:
Stabilization and Transport

Objectives:

Upon completion of this chapter, the physician will be able to define and outline general principles for the **optimal** stabilization and **most appropriate** transportation of trauma patients.

Specifically, the physician will be able to:

A. Identify injuries that may require transfer of trauma patients from a primary care institution to a facility providing a higher level of trauma care.

B. Outline procedures to **optimally** stabilize the trauma patient and prepare him for safe transport to a higher-level trauma care facility.

**Chapter 12:
Stabilization
and
Transport**

I. Introduction

This course is designed to train the students to be more proficient in their ability to stabilize and prepare the patient for definitive care. If definitive care cannot be rendered at the local hospital, the patient will require transfer to a hospital better suited to his needs. Ideally this facility should be an **appropriately** designated trauma center, the level of which will depend on the patient's needs. The decision to transfer the patient to another facility will depend upon the victim's injuries, and the ability of the patient's physician and the local hospital and personnel to care for those injuries. Decisions as to which patients should be transferred, and when, are matters of medical judgment. Recent evidence supports the view that trauma outcome is enhanced if critically injured patients are cared for in facilities prepared for and dedicated to the needs of the acutely injured. **No longer should the patient be transferred to the closest hospital, but rather to the closest appropriate hospital, preferably a designated trauma center.**

The primary principle of trauma management is to **do no further harm.** Indeed, care of the trauma victim should consistently improve with each step, from the scene of the accident to the facility that can provide the patient with the necessary, proper treatment. All those who care for trauma patients must ensure that the level of care never declines from one step to another.

II. Determining the Need for Patient Transfer

The vast majority of patients will receive their total care in the local hospital, and movement beyond that point will not be necessary. However, certain patients will have injuries of such magnitude that facilities and personnel are required beyond those locally available. **It is essential that physicians assess their own capabilities and limitations, and those of their institution, such that they can recognize these patients early and arrange for their transfer to an institution that can provide optimal care.** Once the need for transfer is recognized, arrangements should be expedited, and not delayed for laboratory and roentgenographic examinations or procedures (ie, peritoneal lavage) that do not change the immediate plan of care.

The timing of interhospital transfer will vary based on the distance of transfer, the available skill levels for transfer, circumstances of the local institution, and intervention that is necessary before the patient can be safely transferred. Injuries that can be stabilized, operatively or nonoperatively, by the local institution **must** be treated prior to transport. This treatment may require certain elements of surgical intervention, such as abdominal exploration for control of hemorrhage, to ensure that the patient is in the best possible condition for transfer. Intervention prior to transfer is a **surgical decision** if a surgeon is available locally.

To help the physician determine **which** patients might need care at a higher-level facility, the ACS Committee on Trauma recommends using certain interhospital triage criteria, physiologic parameters, and historical information, ie, concurrent mechanisms of injury or circumstances surrounding the accident. These factors also help the physician decide which stable patients might benefit from transfer. Individuals with certain anatomical injuries or combinations of injuries are in the highest-risk group for mortality, and require a more specialized level of care for optimal recovery. Ideally, such patients should be treated in a facility capable of delivering the highest level of trauma care.

A. Interhospital Triage Criteria

Table 1 (modified from Appendix F–Trauma Decision Scheme and Interhospital Triage Criteria, ACS Hospital Resource Document) identifies patients who are at particularly high risk of dying from multiple and severe injuries. Ideally, such patients should be treated in an institution offering the most specialized trauma care available to ensure optimal outcome. Such patients should be considered for transfer whenever appropriate and possible.

B. Physiological Criteria

Individuals at the extremes of age exhibit physiologic differences which increase the risk of mortality from trauma. Children are at risk for hypothermia and occult visceral injuries. The elderly often have associated medical conditions and use medications that may adversely affect their response to trauma.

Some physiological measurements indicate the need for highly specialized trauma care. These measurements refer to the Glasgow Coma Scale (GCS), systolic blood pressure, and respiratory rate.

The patient who exhibits a Glasgow Coma Score of less than 13, or a deteriorating GCS, is a candidate for transport to a more specialized center.

The patient who persistently exhibits a systolic blood pressure of less than 90 mmHg with resuscitation, is likely to be hemodynamically unstable, and/or continuing to hemorrhage. Such a patient would benefit by transport to a more specialized center.

Patients exhibiting a respiratory rate of less than 10/minute or more than 29/minute may have central nervous system or pulmonary injuries indicating progressive instability, and/or implying serious central nervous system or thoracic injury which will require surgical intervention or ventilatory care. These patients are known to benefit from more specialized trauma care.

C. Circumstances and Mechanism of Injury

Occasionally, patients have few complaints, and appear stable and unhurt when first seen in the emergency department. Under these circumstances, many trauma patients will not have major injuries. However, some may be unaware of the seriousness of their injuries, and will unintentionally mislead the examining physician. Circumstances surrounding the injury event and mechanisms of injury can help alert the physician to possible serious injury.

The victim who walks away from a high-speed crash may be just lucky, or may be harboring occult injuries. Certain events should arouse suspicion that a severe injury may be present, regardless of initial signs. Any patient involved in a vehicular crash in which another occupant of the car was killed should be **thoroughly evaluated** in the hospital for manifestations of occult injury. Epidural hematoma, pancreatic transection, and aortic rupture are examples of injury that may not be recognized initially.

Alcohol and drug abuse are common to all forms of trauma and are particularly important to identify. Physicians should recognize that alcohol and drugs can alter pain perception and mask significant physical findings. Alterations in the patient's responsiveness may be related to alcohol and drugs, but absence of cerebral injury should never be assumed in the presence of alcohol or drugs. If the examining physician is unsure, transfer to a higher level facility may be appropriate.

The mechanism of injury may also suggest to the physician that the patient is at high risk for injury, despite apparent trivial complaints. Deceleration from high speeds, falls from great heights, and close proximity to blast forces are examples of mechanisms of injury that place the patient in a high-risk category. These patients may be initially stable, but their condition can deteriorate rapidly.

III. Transfer Responsibilities

A. Referring Physician

The referring and receiving physicians share the responsibility for patient transfer. The referring physician has the responsibility for initiating patient transfer. Both physicians should communicate directly to ensure that the receiving facility can provide the necessary level of care. Before considering patient transfer the referring physician should have completed the primary and secondary surveys, and instituted measures of resuscitation and stabilization.

B. Receiving Physician

The referring and receiving physicians should consult regarding arrangements and details of patient transfer, including the method of transportation. The physician arranging transportation is responsible for determining what additional care is required before patient transfer, and what capabilities should be available en route.

Remember, the patient requiring transfer to another facility usually has suffered one or more major injuries. Incomplete resuscitation, inadequate stabilization, and absence of transfer data adversely affect patient outcome.

The quality of care rendered en route is also of vital importance to the patient's outcome. Only by direct communication between the referring and receiving physicians can the details of patient transfer be clearly delineated. If adequately trained ambulance personnel are not available, a nurse or physician should accompany the patient.

Table 1

Interhospital Triage Criteria

(Modified from Appendix F—ACS Hospital Resource Document)

Central Nervous System

Head injury   – Penetrating injury or depressed skull fracture
                – Open injury with or without CSF leak
                – Severe injury (GCS < 10) or GCS deterioration
                – Lateralizing signs

Spinal cord injury

Chest

Wide superior mediastinum
Major chest wall injury
Cardiac injury
Patients who may require protracted ventilation

Pelvis

Pelvic ring disruption with shock and evidence of continuing hemorrhage, and open pelvic injury or pelvic visceral injury.

Multiple System Injury

Severe face injury with head injury
Chest injury with head injury
Abdominal or pelvic injury with head injury
Burns with head injury

Evidence of High Energy Impact

Auto crash or pedestrian injury–25 mph or more
Rearward displacement of front axle or front of car (20 inches)
Ejection of patient, or rollover
Death of occupant in same car

Comorbid Factors

Age < 5 years, or > 55 years
Known cardiorespiratory disease

Secondary Deterioration (late sequelae)

Mechanical ventilation required
Sepsis
Single or multiple organ system failure (deterioration in CNS, cardiac, pulmonary, hepatic, renal, or coagulation systems)
Osteomyelitis

Since the transport phase may be the most hazardous phase of care for the trauma patient, air transport—either fixed wing or helicopter—should be seriously considered where available and where weather conditions allow safe transport. Air ambulance systems are expeditious and generally offer high-quality care during transport.

IV. Transfer Protocols

Where protocols for patient transfer do not exist, the following guidelines are suggested.

A. Referring Physician

The local physician wishing to transfer the patient should speak directly to the physician accepting the patient at the receiving hospital, and provide this information:

1. Identification of the patient.

2. A brief history of the incident, including pertinent prehospital data.

3. Initial patient findings, in the emergency department, and the patient's response to the therapy administered.

B. Information to Transferring Personnel

Information regarding the patient's condition and needs during transfer should be communicated to the transporting personnel. This information should include, but not be limited to:

1. Airway maintenance.

2. Fluid volume replacement.

3. Special procedures that may be necessary.

4. Trauma Score, resuscitation procedures, and any changes which may be required en route.

C. Documentation

A written record of the problem, treatment given, and patient status at the time of transfer, as well as certain physical items must accompany the patient. These should include:

1. Initial diagnostic impression.

2. Patient's name, address, hospital number, age; and name, address, and phone number of next of kin.

3. History of injury or illness.

4. Condition on admission.

5. Vital signs prehospital, during stay in emergency department, and at time of transfer.

6. Treatment rendered, including medications given and route of administration.

7. Laboratory and roentgenographic findings, appropriate laboratory specimens (ie, lavage), and all roentgenograms.

8. Fluids given by type and volume.

9. Name, address, and phone number of the referring physician.

10. Name of physician at the receiving institution who has been contacted about the patient.

D. Prior to Transfer

The patient should be resuscitated and attempts made to stabilize his or her condition as completely as possible based on this suggested outline.

1. Respiratory

a. Insert an airway or endotracheal tube, if needed.

b. Determine rate and method of administration of oxygen.

c. Provide suction.

d. Provide mechanical ventilation when needed.

e. Insert a chest tube if needed.

f. Insert a nasogastric tube to prevent aspiration.

2. Cardiovascular

a. Control external bleeding.

b. Establish two large-bore IV lines and begin crystalloid solution infusion.

c. Restore blood volume losses with crystalloid or blood, and continue replacement during transfer.

d. Insert an indwelling catheter to monitor urinary output.

3. Central nervous system

a. Controlled hyperventilation for head-injury patients.

b. Administer mannitol, diuretics, or steroids, if needed, after neurosurgical consultation.

c. Immobilize head, thoracic, and/or lumbar spine injuries.

4. Diagnostic studies as indicated

a. Roentgenogram of the cervical spine.

b. Roentgenogram of the chest.

c. Roentgenogram of the pelvis.

  d. Roentgenogram of the extremities.

  e. Hemoglobin, hematocrit, and arterial blood gases.

  f. Electrocardiogram.

  g. Urinalysis.

5. Wounds

  a. Clean and dress.

  b. Tetanus toxoid.

  c. Tetanus Immune Globulin, if indicated.

  d. Antibiotics, when indicated.

6. Fractures

  a. Appropriate splinting and traction.

  b. Backboard, where indicated.

E. Management During Transport

  1. Continued support of cardiorespiratory system.

  2. Continued blood volume replacement.

  3. Monitoring of vital signs.

  4. Use of appropriate medications as ordered by a physician or as provided by written protocol.

  5. Maintain communication with a physician or institution during the transfer.

  6. Maintain accurate records during transfer.

V. Transfer Data

The information accompanying the patient should **always** include both demographic and historical information pertinent to the patient's injury. In addition to the information already outlined, space should be provided for recording data in an organized, sequential fashion—specifically vital signs, CNS function, and urinary output.

VI. Summary

A. The initial principle of trauma management is to do no further harm.

B. The treating physician should know his or her capabilities and the indications for transfer.

C. The referring physician and receiving physician should communicate directly.

D. Transfer personnel should be adequately skilled to administer the required patient care en route.

Bibliography

1. American College of Surgeons Committee on Trauma: Hospital and Prehospital Resources for Optimal Care of the Injured Patient. 1987.

2. Appendix C to Hospital Resources Document, InterHospital Transfer of Patients. Ibid.

3. Appendix F to Hospital Resources Document, Field Categorization of Trauma Patients. Ibid.

4. Appendix G to Hospital Resources Document, Quality Assurance in Trauma Care. Ibid.

Appendices to Section I
Table of Contents

Appendices

Appendix A:
Ocular Trauma
(Optional Lecture)

Objectives:

Upon completion of this topic the physician will be able to:

A. Obtain patient and event histories.

B. Perform a systematic examination of the orbit and its contents.

C. Identify and discuss those eyelid injuries that can be treated by the primary care physician, and those that must be referred to an ophthalmologist for treatment.

D. Discuss how to examine the eye for a foreign body, and how to remove superficial foreign bodies to prevent further injury.

E. Identify a corneal abrasion, and discuss its management.

F. Identify a hyphema, and discuss the initial management and necessity for referral to an ophthalmologist.

G. Identify those eye injuries requiring referral to an ophthalmologist.

H. Identify a ruptured globe injury, and discuss the initial management required prior to referral to an ophthalmologist.

I. Evaluate and treat eye injuries resulting from chemicals.

J. Evaluate a patient with an orbital fracture, and discuss the initial management and necessity for referral.

K. Identify a retrobulbar hematoma, and discuss the necessity for immediate referral.

**Appendix A:
Ocular
Trauma**

**(Optional
Lecture)**

I. Introduction

The initial assessment of a patient with ocular injury requires a systematic approach. The physical examination should proceed in an organized, step-by-step manner, and does not require extensive, complicated instrumentation in the multiple trauma setting. Simple therapeutic measures often can save the patient's vision and prevent severe sequelae before an ophthalmologist is available. This optional lecture provides that pertinent information about early identification and treatment of ocular injuries that enhances the physician's basic knowledge, and may save the patient's sight.

II. Assessment

A. History

Obtain a history of any pre-existing ocular disease.

1. Does the patient wear corrective lenses?

2. Is there a history of glaucoma?

3. What medications does the patient use, ie, pilocarpine?

B. Injury Incident

Obtain a detailed description of the circumstances surrounding the injury. This information often raises the index of suspicion for certain potential injuries and their sequelae, ie, the higher risk of infection from certain foreign bodies—wood versus metallic.

1. Was there blunt trauma?

2. Was there penetrating injury? In motor vehicular accidents there is potential for glass or metallic foreign bodies.

3. Was there a missile injury?

4. Was there a possible thermal, chemical, or flash burn?

C. Initial Symptoms/Complaint

1. What were the patient's initial symptoms?

2. Did the patient complain of pain or photophobia?

3. Was there an immediate decrease in vision that has remained stable, or is it progressive?

The physical examination must be systematic so that function as well as anatomic structures are evaluated. As with injuries to other organ systems, the pathology also may evolve with time, and the patient must be periodically re-evaluated. A directed approach to the ocular examination, beginning with the most external structures in an "outside-to-inside" manner, ensures that injuries will not be missed.

D. Visual Acuity

Visual acuity is evaluated first by any means possible and recorded, ie, patient counting fingers at three feet.

E. Eyelids

The most external structures to be examined are the eyelids. The eyelids should be assessed for edema; ecchymosis; evidence of burns or chemical injury; laceration(s)—medial, lateral, lid margin, canaliculi; ptosis; foreign bodies that contact the globe; and avulsion of the canthal tendon.

F. Orbital Rim

Gently palpate the orbital rim for a step-off deformity and crepitus. Subcutaneous emphysema may result from a fracture of the medial orbit into the ethmoids, or a fracture of the orbital floor into the maxillary antrum.

G. Globe

The eyelids should be retracted to examine the globe without applying pressure to the globe. The globe is then assessed anteriorly for displacement resulting from a retrobulbar hematoma, and for posterior or inferior displacement due to a fracture of the orbit. The globes are also assessed for normal ocular movement, diplopia at the extremes of the patient's gaze, and evidence of entrapment.

H. Pupil

The pupils are assessed for roundness with regular shape, equality, and reaction to light stimulus.

I. Cornea

The cornea is assessed for opacity, ulceration, and foreign bodies. Fluoroscein and a blue light facilitate this assessment.

J. Conjunctiva

The conjunctivae are assessed for chemosis, subconjunctival emphysema (indicating probable fracture of the orbit into the ethmoid or maxillary sinus), subconjunctival hemorrhage, and nonimpaled foreign bodies.

K. Anterior Chamber

Examine the anterior chamber for a hyphema (blood in the anterior chamber). The depth of the anterior chamber can be assessed by shining a light into the eye from the lateral aspect of the eye. If the light does not illuminate the entire surface of the iris, a shallow anterior chamber should be suspected. A shallow anterior chamber may result from an anterior penetrating wound. A deep anterior chamber may result from a posterior penetrating wound of the globe.

L. Iris

The iris should be regular in shape and reactive. Assess the iris for iridodialysis, a tear of the iris or iridodensis, and a floppy or tremulous iris.

M. Lens

The lens should be transparent. Assess the lens for possible anterior displacement into the anterior chamber, partial dislocation with displacement into the posterior chamber, and dislocation into the vitreous.

N. Vitreous

The vitreous should also be transparent, allowing for easy visualization of the fundus and retina. Visualization may be difficult if vitreous hemorrhage has occurred. In this situation, a black rather than red reflex is seen by ophthalmoscopy. A vitreous bleed usually indicates a significant underlying ocular injury. The vitreous should also be assessed for an intraocular foreign body.

O. Retina

The retina is examined for hemorrhage, possible tears, or detachment. A detached retina is opalescent, and the blood columns are darker.

III. Specific Injuries

A. Lid

Lid injuries often result in marked ecchymosis, making examination of the globe difficult. However, a more serious injury to the underlying structures must be ruled out. Look beneath the lid as well to rule out damage to the globe. Lid retractors should be used if necessary to forcibly open the eye to inspect the globe. Ptosis may be secondary to edema, damage to the levator palpebrae, or oculomotor nerve injury.

Lacerations of the upper lid that are horizontal, superficial, and do not involve the levator may be closed by the examining physician, using five (6-0 to 8-0 silk) sutures. The physician also should examine the eye beneath the lid to rule out damage to the globe.

Lid injuries to be treated by an ophthalmologist include: 1) wounds involving the medial canthus that may have damaged the medial canaliculus; 2) injury to the lacrimal sac or nasal lacrimal duct, which can lead to obstruction if not properly repaired; 3) deep horizontal lacerations of the upper lid that may involve the levator, and result in ptosis if not repaired correctly; and 4) lacerations of the lid margin that are difficult to close, and may lead to notching, entropion, or ectropion.

Foreign bodies of the lid result in profuse tearing, pain, and a foreign-body sensation that increases with lid movement. The conjunctiva should be injected, and the upper and lower lids everted to examine the inner surface. Topical anesthetic drops may be used, but **only** for initial examination and removal of the foreign body.

Impaled, penetrating foreign bodies are not disturbed, and are removed only in the operating room by an ophthalmologist or appropriate specialist. If the patient requires transport to another facility for treatment of this injury or others, apply a dressing about the foreign body to stabilize it.

B. Cornea

Corneal abrasions result in pain, foreign body sensation, photophobia, decreasing visual acuity, and chemosis. The injured epithelium stains with fluoroscein.

Corneal foreign bodies sometimes can be removed with irrigation. However, if the foreign body is embedded, the patient should be referred. Corneal foreign bodies are treated with antibiotic drops or ointment (eg, sulfacetamide or neomycin combination, bacitracin, or polymyxin). The eye should then be patched to prevent movement, minimize pain, and promote faster healing in the case of an abrasion, or prevent further injury if there is an embedded foreign body. Patients with embedded foreign bodies should be referred to an ophthalmologist.

C. Anterior Chamber

Hyphema is blood in the anterior chamber, which may be difficult to see if there is only a small amount of blood. In extreme cases, the entire anterior chamber is filled. The hyphema can often be seen with a pen light. Hyphema usually indicates severe intraocular trauma.

Seven percent of patients with hyphema develop glaucoma. Corneal staining may also occur. **Remember**, hyphema may be the result of serious underlying ocular injury. Even in the case of small bleed, spontaneous rebleeding often occurs within the first five days, which may lead to total hyphema. Therefore, the patient must be referred. Both eyes are patched, the patient is usually hospitalized, placed at bed rest, and re-evaluated frequently. Pain after hyphema usually indicates rebleeding and/or acute glaucoma.

D. Iris

Contusion injuries of the iris may cause traumatic mydriasis or miosis. There may be a disruption of the iris from the ciliary body, causing an irregular pupil and hyphema.

E. Lens

Contusion of the lens may lead to later opacification. Blunt trauma can cause a break of the zonular fibers that encircle the lens and anchor it to the ciliary body. This results in subluxation of the lens, possibly into the anterior chamber, causing a shallow chamber and acute, closed-angle glaucoma. In cases of posterior subluxation, the anterior chamber deepens. Patients with this injury should be referred to an ophthalmologist.

F. Vitreous

Blunt trauma can also lead to vitreous hemorrhage. This is usually secondary to retinal vessel damage and bleeding into the vitreous, resulting in a sudden, profound visual loss. Fundoscopic exam may be impossible, and the red reflex, seen with an ophthalmoscope light, is lost. A patient with this injury should be placed at bed rest with binocular patches and referred to an ophthalmologist.

G. Retina

Blunt trauma also causes retinal hemorrhage. The patient may or may not have decreased visual acuity, depending on involvement of the macula. Superficial retinal hemorrhages appear cherry red in color; the deeper lesions, gray.

Retinal edema and detachment can occur with head trauma. A white, cloudy discoloration is observed. Retinal detachments appear "curtain-like." If the macula is involved, visual acuity is affected. An acute retinal tear usually occurs in conjunction with blunt trauma to an eye with pre-existing vitreoretinal pathology. Retinal detachment most often occurs as a late sequela of blunt trauma. The patient describes light flashes and a curtain-like defect in peripheral vision.

A rupture of the choroid (blood supply of the retina) initially appears as a beige area at the posterior pole. Later it becomes a yellow-white scar. If it transects the macula, vision is seriously and permanently impaired.

H. Globe

A patient with a ruptured globe has marked visual impairment. The eye is soft due to a decreased intraocular pressure, and the anterior chamber is flattened or shallow. If the rupture is anterior, ocular contents may be seen extruding from the eye.

The goal of initial management of the ruptured globe is to protect the eye from any additional damage. A sterile dressing and eye shield should be carefully applied to prevent any pressure to the eye that may cause further extrusion of the ocular contents. The patient should be instructed not to squeeze his eye shut. If not contraindicated by other injuries, the patient may be sedated while awaiting transport or treatment. Do not remove foreign objects, tissue, or clots before dressing placement. No topical analgesics are used—only oral or parenteral, if not contraindicated by any other injuries.

An intraocular foreign body should be suspected if the patient complains of sudden sharp pain with a decrease in visual acuity. Inspect the surface of the globe carefully for any small lacerations and possible sites of entry. These may be difficult to find. In the anterior chamber, tiny foreign bodies may be hidden by blood or in the crypts of the iris. A tiny iris perforation may be impossible to see directly, but with a pen light the red reflex may be detected through the defect (if the lens and vitreous are not opaque).

I. Chemical Injuries

Chemical injuries require immediate intervention if sight is to be preserved. Acid precipitates proteins in the tissue and sets up somewhat of a natural barrier against extensive tissue penetration. However, alkali combines with lipids in the cell membrane, leading to disruption of the cell membranes, rapid penetration of the caustic agent, and extensive tissue destruction. Chemical injury of the cornea causes disruption of stromal mucopolysaccharidea, leading to opacification.

The treatment is **copious and continuous irrigation**. Attempts should not be made to neutralize the agent. Intravenous solutions (sterile saline or Ringer's lactate) and tubing can be used to improvise continuous irrigation. Blepharospasm is extensive, and the lids must be manually opened during irrigation. Analgesics and sedation should be used, if not contraindicated by coexisting injuries.

Thermal injuries usually occur to the lids only and rarely involve the cornea. However, burns of the globe occasionally occur. A sterile dressing should be applied and the patient referred to an ophthalmologist. Exposure of the cornea **must** be prevented, or it can perforate, and the eye can be lost.

J. Fracture

Blunt trauma to the orbit causes rapid compression of the tissues and increased pressure within the orbit. The weakest point is the orbital floor, which fractures, allowing the periorbital fat and possibly the inferior rectus and/or inferior oblique muscles to herniate into the antrum—hence the term, "blow out" fracture.

Clinically the patient presents with pain, swelling, and ecchymosis of the lids and periorbital tissues. There may be subconjunctival hemorrhage. Facial asymmetry and possibly enophthalmos might be evident or masked by surrounding edema. Limitation of ocular motion and diplopia secondary to edema or entrapment of extraocular muscles may be noted. Palpation of the infraorbital rim often reveals a step-off. Subcutaneous and/or subconjunctival emphysema can occur when the fracture is into the ethmoid or maxillary sinuses. Hypesthesias of the cheek occur secondary to injury of the infraorbital nerve.

The Waters view and Caldwell view (straight on) are very helpful for evaluating orbital fractures. Examine the orbital floor, and look for soft tissue density in the maxillary sinus or an air fluid level (blood). CT scans are also helpful, and may be considered mandatory.

Exophthalmometry must be performed as son as possible. Treatment of fractures may be delayed up to a week. If entrapment is suspected, a forced duction test should be performed. (The inferior rectus is grasped with a forceps to test for entrapment.) Watchful waiting has avoided unnecessary surgery by allowing the edema to decrease, allowing more accurate evaluation of the cosmetic or functional deficit.

J. Retrobulbar Hematoma

A retrobulbar hematoma requires immediate treatment by an ophthalmologist. The resulting increased pressure within the orbit compromises the blood supply to the retina and optic nerve, resulting in blindness if not treated.

K. Fat Emboli

Patients with long-bone fractures are at risk for fat emboli. Remember, this is a possible cause of sudden change in vision for a patient who has sustained multiple injuries.

IV. Summary

Thorough, systematic evaluation of the injured eye results in few significant injuries being missed. Once the injuries have been identified, treat the eye injury using simple measures, prevent further damage, and help preserve sight until the patient is in the ophthalmologist's care.

Appendix B:
Pediatric Triage and Injury Scoring

Pediatric Trauma Score

PTS	+2	+1	-1
Weight	> 44 lbs (> 20 kg)	22-44 lbs (10-20 kg)	< 22 lbs (< 10 kg)
Airway	Normal	Oral or nasal airway	Intubated, tracheostomy invasive
Blood pressure	> 90 mmHg	50-90 mmHg	< 50 mmHg
Level of consciousness	Completely awake	Obtunded or any LOC*	Comatose
Open wound	None	Minor	Major or penetrating
Fractures	None	Minor	Open or multiple fractures
TOTALS:			

*Loss of consciousness

**Appendix B:
Pediatric
Triage and
Injury
Scoring**

Pediatric Triage and Injury Scoring

The tragedy of preventable traumatic death has been well documented in multiple studies over the past three decades. Studies of the pediatric population show an incidence of 53 out of 100 pediatric trauma deaths that could be classified as preventable. These statistics have been one of the prime motivating factors for developing regional trauma referral systems, intended to provide continuous, high-quality, sophisticated care in a few specifically designated care centers.

Because this level of care and commitment is extremely expensive, the functional efficiency of such systems depends on accurate and judicious triage of injured patients to appropriately designated centers. This problem becomes even more acute for pediatric trauma patients, because the few hospitals that are designated as pediatric trauma centers frequently serve relatively large, broad population areas. Intelligent triage thus becomes a major factor, not only in the determination of initial care, but also in the overall function of and impact on the regional trauma system.

The Pediatric Trauma Score (PTS) was developed specifically as a triage tool for pediatric trauma victims. This grading system assesses and assigns a value to each of six components of pediatric injury. These values are added to arrive at a score that predicts injury severity and potential for mortality.

Size is considered first because it is obvious, and is a major consideration for the infant-toddler group, in which mortality from injury is the highest. **Airway** is assessed not just as a function, but as a descriptor of what care is required to provide adequate management. **Systolic blood pressure** assessment primarily identifies those children in whom evolving, preventable shock may occur [50 to 90 mmHg systolic blood pressure (+1)]. Regardless of size, a child whose systolic blood pressure is below 50 mmHg (-1) is in obvious jeopardy. On the other hand, a child whose systolic pressure exceeds 90 mmHg (+2) probably falls into a better outcome category than a child with even a slight degree of hypotension.

Level of consciousness is the most important factor in initially assessing the central nervous system. Because children frequently lose consciousness transiently during injury, the "obtunded" (+1) grade is given to any child who loses consciousness, no matter how fleeting the loss. This grade identifies a patient who may have sustained a head injury with potentially fatal—but often treatable—intracranial sequelae.

Skeletal injury is also a component of the PTS, because of its high incidence in the pediatric population and its potential contribution to mortality. Finally, **cutaneous injury,** both as an adjunct to common pediatric injury patterns and as an injury category that includes penetrating wounds, is considered in the computed PTS.

The PTS serves as a simple checklist, ensuring that all components critical to initial assessment of the injured child have been considered. It is useful for paramedics in the field, as well as for physicians in facilities other than pediatric trauma units. As a predictor of injury, the PTS has a statistically significant inverse relationship with the Injury Severity Score (ISS) and mortality. Analysis of this relationship has identified a threshold PTS of eight, below which all injured children should be triaged to an appropriate pediatric trauma center. These children have the highest potential for preventable mortality and morbidity. According to the National Pediatric Trauma Registry statistics, they represent approximately 25% of all pediatric trauma victims, clearly requiring the most aggressive monitoring and observation.

Appendix C:
Tetanus Immunization

Introduction

Attention must be directed to adequate tetanus prophylaxis in the multiply injured patient, particularly if open-extremity trauma is present. Tetanus immunization depends on the patient's previous immunization status and the tetanus-prone nature of the wound. The following guidelines have been adapted from *A Guide to Prophylaxis Against Tetanus in Wound Management,* prepared by the ACS Committee on Trauma. Because this information is reviewed and updated as new data become available, the Committee on Trauma recommends contacting the Center for Disease Control for the latest information and detailed guidelines related to tetanus prophylaxis and immunization for the injured patient.

I. General Principles

A. Individual Assessment

The attending physician must determine the requirements for adequate prophylaxis against tetanus for each injured patient individually.

B. Surgical Wound Care

Regardless of the active immunization status of the patient, meticulous surgical care—including removal of all devitalized tissue and foreign bodies—should be provided immediately for all wounds. Such care is essential as part of the prophylaxis against tetanus; it is the basis of definitive surgical management. However, such treatment must be instituted as soon as possible. Therefore, minimal delay in definitive care is indicated.

C. Human Tetanus Immune Globulin (TIG)

Passive immunization with 250 units of Tetanus Immune Globulin (TIG), administered intramuscularly, must be considered individually for each patient. TIG provides longer protection than antitoxin of animal origin and causes few adverse reactions. The characteristics of the wound, conditions under which it occurred, its age, TIG treatment, and the previous active immunization status of the patient must be considered (Table 2). When tetanus toxoid and TIG are given concurrently, separate syringes and separate sites should be used.

If the patient has ever received two or more injections of toxoid, TIG is not indicated, unless the wound is judged to be tetanus-prone and is more than 24 hours old. Do not administer equine tetanus antitoxin, except when the human antitoxin is not available, and only if the possibility of tetanus outweighs the potential reactions of horse serum.

D. Documentation

For every injured patient, information about the mechanism of injury, the characteristics of the wound, age, previous active immunization status, history of a neurologic or severe hypersensitivity reaction following a previous immunization treatment, and plans for follow-up should be documented. Each patient must be given a written record describing treatment rendered, and follow-up instructions that outline wound care, drug therapy, immunization status, and potential complications. The patient should be referred to a designated physician who will provide comprehensive follow-up care, including completion of active immunizations.

A wallet-sized card documenting the immunization administered and date of immunization should be given to every injured patient. The patient should be instructed to carry the written record at all times, and complete active immunization, if indicated. For precise tetanus prophylaxis, an accurate and immediately available history regarding previous active immunization against tetanus is required. Otherwise, rapid laboratory titration is necessary to determine the patient's serum antitoxin level.

E. Antibiotics

The effectiveness of antibiotics for prophylaxis of tetanus is uncertain. Proper immunization plays the most important role in tetanus prophylaxis.

F. Contraindications

The only contraindication to tetanus and diphtheria toxoids in the wounded patient is a history of neurologic or severe hypersensitivity reaction following a previous dose. Local side effects alone do not preclude continued use. If a systemic reaction is suspected to represent allergic hypersensitivity, immunization should be postponed until appropriate skin testing is undertaken at a later time. If a tetanus toxoid-containing preparation is contraindicated, passive immunization against tetanus should be considered for a tetanus-prone wound.

Contraindications to pertussis vaccination in infants and children less than seven years old include either a previous adverse reaction after DTP or single-antigen pertussis vaccination, and/or the presence of a neurologic finding. If such a contraindication to using pertussis vaccine adsorbed (P) exists, diphtheria and tetanus toxoid adsorbed (for pediatric use) (DT) is recommended. A static neurologic condition, such as cerebral palsy, or a family history of convulsions or other central nervous system disorders, is not a contraindication to giving vaccines containing the pertussis antigen.

G. Active Immunization for Normal Infants and Children

For children under seven years of age, immunization requires four injections of diphtheria and tetanus toxoids and pertussis vaccine adsorbed (DTP). A booster (fifth dose) injection is administered at four to six years of age. Thereafter, a routine booster of tetanus and diphtheria toxoids adsorbed (Td) is indicated at ten-year intervals (for adult use).

H. Active Immunization for Adults

Immunization for adults requires at least three injections of Td. An injection of Td should be repeated every ten years throughout the individual's life, providing no significant reactions to Td have occurred.

I. Active Immunization for Pregnant Women

Neonatal tetanus is preventable by active immunization of the pregnant mother during the first six months of pregnancy, with two injections of Td given two months apart. After delivery and six months after the second dose, the mother should be given the third dose of Td to complete the active immunization.

An injection of Td should be repeated every ten years throughout life, providing no significant reactions to Td have occurred. In the event that a neonate is born to a nonimmunized mother without obstetric care, the infant should receive 250 units of TIG. Active and passive immunization of the mother should also be initiated.

J. Previously Immunized Individuals

1. Fully immunized

When the attending physician has determined that the patient has been previously and fully immunized, and the last dose of toxoid was given **within ten years**:

a. Administer 0.5 ml adsorbed toxoid for tetanus-prone wounds, if more than five years has elapsed since the last dose.

b. This booster may be omitted if excessive toxoid injections have been given before.

2. Partially immunized

When the patient has received two or more injections of toxoid, and the last dose was received **more than ten years ago, 0.5 ml adsorbed toxoid is administered** for both tetanus-prone and nontetanus-prone wounds. Passive immunization is not necessary.

K. Individuals Not Adequately Immunized

When the patient has received **only one or no** prior injections of toxoid, or the immunization history is unknown:

1. Nontetanus-prone wounds

Administer 0.5 ml of adsorbed toxoid for nontetanus-prone wounds.

2. Tetanus-prone wounds

a. Administer 0.5 ml adsorbed toxoid.

b. Administer 250 units TIG.

c. Consider administering antibiotics, although their effectiveness for prophylaxis of tetanus remains unproven.

d. Administer medications using different syringes and sites for injection.

L. Immunization Schedule

1. Adult

a. Three injections of toxoid.

b. Booster every ten years.

2. Children

a. Four injections DPT.

b. Fifth dose at four to six years of age.

c. Booster every ten years.

II. Specific Measures for Patients with Wounds

Recommendations for tetanus prophylaxis are based on 1) condition of the wound, and 2) the patient's immunization history. Table 1 outlines some of the clinical features of wounds that are prone to develop tetanus. A wound with any one of these features is a tetanus-prone wound.

Table 1

Clinical Features	Nontetanus-prone Wounds	Tetanus-prone Wounds
Age of wound	≤ 6 hours	> 6 hours
Configuration	Linear wound	Stellate wound, avulsion, abrasion
Depth	≤ 1 cm	> 1 cm
Mechanism of injury	Sharp surface (eg, knife, glass)	Missile, crush burn, frostbite
Signs of infection	Absent	Present
Devitalized tissue	Absent	Present
Contaminants (dirt, feces, soil, saliva, etc.)	Absent	Present
Denervated, and/or ischemic tissue	Absent	Present

Table 2

Summary of Tetanus Prophylaxis for the Injured Patient

History of Adsorbed Tetanus Toxoid (doses)	Nontetanus-prone Wounds		Tetanus-prone Wounds	
	Td[1]	TIG	Td[1]	TIG
Unknown or ≤ three	Yes	No	Yes	Yes
≥ three[2]	No[3]	No	No[4]	No

Key to Table 2

1   For children under seven years old: DTP (DT, if pertussis vaccine is contraindicated) is preferred to tetanus toxoid alone. For persons seven years old and older, Td is preferred to tetanus toxoid alone.

2   If only three doses of fluid toxoid have been received, a fourth dose of toxoid, preferably an adsorbed toxoid, should be given.

3   Yes, if more than ten years since last dose.

4   Yes, if more than five years since last dose. (More frequent boosters are not needed and can accentuate side effects.)

Td   Tetanus and diphtheria toxoids adsorbed—for adult use

TIG   Tetanus Immune Globulin—Human

American College of Surgeons

Appendix D:
Preparations for Disaster

Introduction

These guidelines for disaster preparation were adapted directly from *Early Care of the Injured Patient*, by the Committee on Trauma of the American College of Surgeons, Alexander J. Walt, MD (Editor), 1982, "Disaster Planning for Mass Casualties," Chapter 24, page 377.

Appendix D:
Preparations
for
Disaster

I. Planning and Preparation

Disaster planning, whether at the state, regional, or local level, involves a wide-range of individuals and resources. **All plans:**

A. Should involve high-level officials of the local police, fire, and civil defense agencies.

B. Must be written and tested (at least twice a year) in advance.

C. Must provide for communication arrangements, taking into account the likely overtaxing of existing telephone systems. Designated telephone lines inside and outside the hospital, and portable radio receivers obviate the need for routing messages through switchboards, which by the nature of the situation are almost certain to become overtaxed.

D. Must provide for storage of special equipment and supplies.

E. Must provide for routine first aid.

F. Must provide for definitive care.

G. Must prepare for transfer of casualties to other facilities by prior agreement, should the location in question be overtaxed or unusable.

H. Must consider the urgent needs of patients already hospitalized for conditions unrelated to the disaster.

II. Hospital Planning

Although a regional approach to planning is ideal for the management of mass casualties, circumstances may require that each hospital function with little or no outside support. Earthquakes, floods, riots, or nuclear contamination may force the individual hospital to function in isolation. The crisis may be instantaneous, as with an explosion, or may develop slowly, as do most civil disturbances, malfunctions of nuclear reactors, and floods. Developments that cannot be predicted may have great influence on preventing access to designated disaster facilities. Once a state of disaster has been declared by civil authorities or internally by the hospital director, specific hospital procedures should be performed automatically. These include:

A. Notification of personnel.

B. Preparation of treatment areas.

C. Classification to differentiate emergency department and hospital patients.

D. Checking of supplies of blood, fluids, medications, food, potable water, and other materials essential to hospital operation.

E. Provision for decontamination procedures, which take high priority in nuclear accidents.

F. Institution of security precautions.

G. Control of visitors and press.

American College of Surgeons

Appendix E:
ATLS and the Law
(Optional Lecture)

Appendix E:
ATLS
and the
Law

(Optional
Lecture)

Objectives:

Upon completion of this topic the student will be able to:

A. Apply practical knowledge of basic medicolegal principles to delivery of trauma patient care.

B. Identify possible sources of liability exposure.

**Appendix E:
ATLS
and the
Law**

**(Optional
Lecture)**

I. Introduction

Appendix E:
ATLS
and the
Law

(Optional
Lecture)

The Committee on Trauma of the American College of Surgeons emphasizes that trauma is a disease of all ages; swift in onset and slow in recovery. Each year accidents disable approximately ten million Americans and kill another 100,000. The ATLS Course is designed to prepare physicians to exercise a quantum of basic knowledge and skills such as rapid assessment, resuscitation, stabilization, appropriate use of consultation, and transfer where necessary.

The overriding principle of the ATLS Course is *primum non nocere;* that is, first do no harm. *Primum non nocere* also implies that a physician who fails to properly exercise advanced trauma life support principles may negligently cause avoidable, unnecessary injury. In the final analysis, the physician must develop "first-hour competence," which demands the proper exercise of ATLS principles in order to save lives, reduce morbidity, and avoid unnecessary harm.

The ideas behind ATLS enhance societal expectations that many lives will be saved and morbidity will be reduced if the proper techniques are exercised. When societal expectations are enhanced by the advancements and claims of the medical profession, there is a corresponding concern that where unexpected injury occurs, someone may have malpracticed.

Note: This optional lecture is not to be considered legal advice, nor a substitute for advice of counsel. This presentation is an overview of certain areas of the law, and of particular interest to participants in the ATLS program.

II. Objectives of ATLS and the Law

Liability exposure occurs when any physician attempting trauma care fails to exercise that degree of knowledge, skill, and due care expected of a reasonably competent practitioner in the same class, acting in the same or similar circumstances. This standard of care, particularly applicable to ATLS, will be discussed more completely later in this text.

The objective of "ATLS and the Law" is to provide an understandable, practical, applicable knowledge of basic medicolegal principles. Upon completion, each participant should be able to identify possible sources of liability exposure. **Remember, good medicine is good law.** Physicians need not fear the law when they exercise diligence (attentiveness) and due care (carefulness or caution) during the diagnostic and treatment processes.

III. Medicolegal Principles

The following medicolegal principles are reviewed in this text.

1. Physician/patient relationship
2. Consent
3. Right to refuse treatment
4. Artificial life support
5. Negligence

**Appendix E:
ATLS
and the
Law**

**(Optional
Lecture)**

IV. Physician/Patient Relationship

A. Contract

Mutual consent is the principle applied to the traditional physician/patient relationship. The patient requests diagnosis and treatment; the physician agrees to provide professional services; the patient agrees to pay; the physician accepts a duty to provide appropriate medical care. Ordinarily, recovery for malpractice against a physician is allowed only where an express or implied contractural relationship exists between the physician and the patient. However, the duty of a physician to bring skill and care to the diagnosis and treatment of a patient does not arise out of contract, but out of policy considerations based on the nature of a physician's function.

B. Undertaking to Treat

Situations have arisen in which the traditional contract theory does not seem to apply, yet courts have found that a physician/patient relationship exists by applying the "undertaking to treat" theory. Advanced trauma life support is a specialty to which this theory is particularly appropriate. In many situations, physicians "undertake to treat" by immediately providing emergency medical care in the absence of any mutual assent. Nevertheless, a binding physician/patient relationship begins the moment the physician undertakes the treatment.

1. Telephone

In a well-known New Jersey case, *O'Neill v. Montefiore Hospital,* 202 NY S2d 436 1960, a patient presented to the emergency department of Montefiore Hospital complaining of chest pain. The emergency department physician examined the patient and requested the on-call physician cardiologist to review the case. The cardiologist elected to discuss the case over the telephone with the patient, and decided the patient could go home. One hour later, while disrobing at home, the patient "dropped dead." The patient's estate sued the hospital, the emergency department physician, and the cardiologist. The cardiologist contended that he was not liable because no contract was made with the patient.

The Supreme Court of New Jersey rejected the contention, outlining that the cardiologist had established a physician/patient relationship by discussing the case with the patient via the telephone, and advising the patient to go home.

The morals of this case are: do not talk to patients on the telephone while on call to the emergency department, and do not engage in therapeutic endeavors with unknown patients via the telephone. The physician may be concerned that this admonition would apply to any patient, particularly patients who are well-known to the physician. Even when the patient is known, telephone advice may create liability exposure. The individual physician should consider this factor as part of his medical judgment.

2. Subordinate physician

In another case, *Smart v. Kansas City*, 105 SW 709 (Mo 1907), the chief of orthopedics was searching the outpatient department for teaching materials. He observed one of the residents examining a patient, walked over, examined the patient, and advised the resident to amputate below the knee. The resident did and committed malpractice. The patient sued the hospital, the resident, and the chief of orthopedics. The chief of orthopedics contended that he was not liable because he did not enter into a physician/patient contract. The state supreme court disagreed, stating the chief of orthopedics was "in charge," ordered the resident to amputate, and subsequently was responsible for the resident's actions, and indeed had entered into a physician/patient relationship.

3. Medical staff conference

Is a presiding physician at a medical staff conference liable for advising a staff physician during a case presentation, if such advice allegedly leads to medical malpractice? A California court ruled that where a practicing physician seeks advice "from a professor" by presenting a case at a regularly scheduled medical staff conference, the physician, acting as professor, will not be liable. The court reasoned that the professor is not "in control" of the practicing physician's activities, because the physician is free to disregard the professor's advice. Therefore, the plaintiff cannot reach the professor by contending that his physician followed professorial advice. *Rainer v. Grossman*, 31 Cal. App. 3d 539, 107 Cal. Rptr. 469 (2nd Dist., 1973).

4. Gratuitous service

Gratuitous medical care is subject to liability. The mere fact that the physician does not collect a fee does not bar the patient from suing for medical malpractice. Treating a friend's child in the middle of the night creates liability exposure, and the courts will not accept a defense of, "I did it for nothing."

Once a physician gives his medical opinion regarding diagnosis or treatment, directly or indirectly, he places himself in a physician/patient relationship. This relationship also can arise if the actions of the patient and physician imply that such a relationship exists. In such instances, the courts have held that the physician's words or actions have, either directly or indirectly, caused the patient to rely on the opinions or representations of the physician. The physician's duty is not to abandon the case or abdicate his responsibility. He also has a duty to exercise that degree of skill, judgment, knowledge, and concern that would be expected of a reasonably competent medical practitioner acting under the same or similar circumstances.

C. Duty to Rescue

There is no legal duty to rescue another person. However, moral and ethical duties may exist and must be distinguished from legal duties.

**Appendix E:
ATLS
and the
Law**

**(Optional
Lecture)**

1. Moral duty

A moral duty is self-imposed, originating from family and ethnic mores, religious exposure, and personal philosophical principles.

2. Ethical duty

An ethical duty arises from membership in unions, associations, or societies. Such organized groups have ethical standards by which they expect their members to act.

3. Legal duty

A legal duty is imposed by law, which expects a person to behave in a certain manner under certain circumstances. The common law (law of the courts) does not impose a legal duty on a person to rescue another person. Therefore, if a physician encounters a stranger on the street who needs CPR, the law would not impose a duty upon the physician to attempt a rescue. The physician may have difficulty dealing with his ethical and moral duties by refusing to do anything, but the law will not hold him responsible.

In some situations, the law does impose a duty to rescue. For example, if a physician encounters his own patient on the street, and that patient needs CPR, the physician is under legal duty to render emergency care. A parent is under legal duty to rescue his child. A public servant, such as a policeman or fireman, is under legal duty to rescue persons in distress. A lifeguard or physician in a hospital is under legal duty by virtue of his employment to rescue patients. It should be noted that once a person undertakes the rescue, he is under a legal duty to do all he can to complete the rescue without causing injury to himself. However, the law does not expect anyone to lose his own life, even when there is a legal duty to rescue.

D. Good Samaritan Statutes

Good Samaritan statutes exist in every state, not because of any evidence that rescuers have been successfully sued, but to encourage potential rescuers to render aid in an emergency. Several states have mandated a rescue. However, legislative exceptions to the mandate raise a question about the enforceability to such laws, because no one is expected to injure himself, or even stop, if he must attend to matters of greater import.

Physicians and health care providers should not refuse to rescue for fear of legal liability, because the potential for a successful suit is virtually nonexistent unless the physician performs in a grossly or shockingly negligent manner. The following scenario is an example of such gross negligence.

A physician encounters a patient lying in the street who has just been ejected through a car's windshield. He observes that the patient has no apparent breathing or circulatory difficulties, or any signs of external hemorrhage. Yet the physician decides to examine the patient, inadvertently moves the head, and causes the patient to become quadriplegic.

Based on these facts, the physician committed gross negligence. Every physician knows or should know that patients sustaining head injuries may have

**Appendix E:
ATLS
and the
Law**

**(Optional
Lecture)**

a concomitant cervical-spine injury. Conversely, if the same patient had an obstructed airway or hemorrhage requiring immediate treatment to prevent death, and the physician followed the basic principles of ATLS, the physician would not be liable for gross negligence, or even ordinary negligence, because the risk of death was greater than the risk of quadriplegia.

V. Consent

A. Battery

Traditionally, the concept of consent is governed by the law of battery. A person is liable for the tort of battery whenever there is an intentional and unpermitted touching of another person. A person does not have to engage in fisticuffs to commit a battery. The mere intentional touching of a person without consent is a battery. A patient who has specifically consented to a panhysterectomy has not consented to an appendectomy. Patients have successfully sued physicians for battery when an unrequested incidental appendectomy has been performed. Liability in such cases depends on whether the patient has implied consent in some way to the additional procedure.

B. Implied Consent in an Emergency

The law usually presumes consent. In an action for malpractice based on lack of consent, the plaintiff must prove that the physician did not obtain consent. If it is practicable to obtain actual consent for treatment from the patient or someone authorized to consent for him, this must be done. However, in an emergency situation in which immediate action is necessary for the protection of the patient's life, the law will imply consent if it cannot be obtained. The law presumes that most reasonable persons under the same or similar circumstances would want their lives saved, if at all possible. This presumption is generally true even when the patient is not competent to consent for himself, as in the case of a minor or someone under the care of a third party, such as a natural guardian, a legal guardian, or a person whom the law of the state allows to substitute consent for the patient. If the emergency immediately endangers the life or permanent health of the patient, a physician should do what the occasion demands.

C. Consent: Competence and Capacity

A physician must understand the difference between capacity and competence. A fully conscious minor is usually not considered to consent to surgery, even if he understands what is happening. Some states have created exceptions to this rule, but generally his parents must consent for him. However, a competent adult may lack the capacity to consent due to a comatose state. Whether someone lacks the capacity to consent depends on the facts in each case, for courts have even held that an intoxicated adult has the capacity to consent. The general standard given by the courts in cases involving questions of capacity to consent is whether the patient understands the risks involved in consenting to treatment and in refusing to consent to treatment.

Appendix E:
ATLS
and the
Law

(Optional
Lecture)

D. Third-Party Consent

1. Minors

The common-law doctrine is clear in stating that minors cannot consent to treatment unless their parents or natural or legal guardians consent. One parent is usually enough, but some states may require both parents to consent. A number of exceptions to this rule are statutory in nature, governed by state legislative law. Therefore, the state statutes should be reviewed to determine those situations in which a minor can consent without parental permission. Generally, minors may consent without parental permission if they are emancipated, pregnant, seeking contraception, seeking treatment for drug abuse, parents themselves, or married. However, tubal ligation or any type of major surgery usually requires parental consent.

2. Spouses

As a general rule, one spouse cannot exercise consent rights for another spouse. A number of cases emphatically underscore the principle that one spouse cannot interfere with the consent rights of another spouse to undergo treatment, including the right of a woman to have an abortion during the first trimester of pregnancy.

3. Next of kin

The patient's next of kin usually does not have a right to substitute consent for the patient. This is true even though the next of kin is the designee for permission to perform an autopsy on a relative in most states. On July 1, 1984, the state of Maryland passed a law providing that the next of kin may give substitute consent for an incompetent patient under certain circumstances. The new law, however, did not interfere with the established doctrines of consent regarding the competent patient or the patient in the emergency situation. The Maryland law states that the available next of kin, in the following order of preference, may give the necessary consent: 1) the spouse, 2) an adult child, 3) a parent, 4) a sibling, 5) a grandparent, or 6) an adult grandchild. The Maryland law probably represents a trend. The purpose of such laws is to avoid legal entanglements in order to obtain consent to effectively treat an incompetent patient.

4. Family members

In the absence of a legally granted authority or "next-of- kin" substitute-consent statute, the common law does not permit family members to exercise the consent rights of another family member, even if the patient is incompetent.

E. Informed Consent

Most courts emphatically hold that consent to treatment, to be effective, must be informed. Informed consent is rarely an issue during life-saving processes. Acute trauma incapacitates many patients, rendering them incapable of communicating or understanding the emergency treatment. The more urgent the medical situation, the less likely that consent of any kind will be an issue. Therefore, informed consent will not be discussed in detail. Remember,

**Appendix E:
ATLS
and the
Law**

**(Optional
Lecture)**

where the patient or his third-party substitute can give consent, that consent must be based on knowledge and understanding of the treatment to be given, and the risks involved in either undergoing or failing to undergo recommended treatment.

F. Physician Defenses to Lack of Consent

1. Consent implied

The patient's lack of capacity and its effect on consent has already been discussed and is self-evident. A second defense, closely related to the first, is that the consent was implied from the circumstances. The physician may contend that he reasonably inferred that the patient's voluntary submission to the treatment indicated consent. The inference may be drawn only if the patient, or a reasonable person in similar circumstances, should have been aware that this passive submission to an obvious procedure constitutes consent to treatment.

2. Disclosure unduly alarming

Another defense, usually used in cases regarding informed consent, is that the disclosure of information concerning the adverse effects of treatment would unduly alarm a patient. The courts have fashioned this defense for the physician by pointing out that situations arise in which the physician knows the patient would become unduly alarmed when informed of the treatment risks, and would probably reject essential treatment that would reduce morbidity or mortality. In those situations, the physician is generally not liable for failing to obtain fully informed consent.

VI. Right to Refuse Treatment

A. Source of Right

The right to refuse treatment is derived from the common law, the principles of democracy, and the United States Constitution.

1. Common Law

The common-law doctrine states that "every human being of adult years and sound mind has a right to determine what shall be done with his own body; and a (physician who administers treatment) without his patient's consent commits a battery for which he is liable in damages."

2. Democracy

Courts also have used the principles of democracy to enforce the right to refuse treatment. They point out that the American democratic system promises us the implied fundamental right to make choices about our personal existence.

**Appendix E:
ATLS
and the
Law**

**(Optional
Lecture)**

3. Constitution

The right to refuse treatment also arises from the United States Constitution as interpreted by the United States Supreme Court. The Constitution's Bill of Rights promises us freedom of speech, freedom of religion, freedom to assemble, the right against unlawful searches and seizures, the right not to have soldiers housed in our homes during peacetime, and the right against self-incrimination. The U. S. Supreme Court has noted that we have other, unwritten Constitutional guarantees implied from that Bill of Rights. In a number of decisions, the Supreme Court has emphasized the right of privacy and the right against bodily invasion by protecting the right to use and receive contraceptives, the right to marry a person of another race, the right to possess pornographic literature at home, and the right to terminate pregnancy.

The Supreme Court has further pointed out that these rights are not absolute, but are subject to certain specific state interests, which will be discussed later in this text.

B. Right of Self-Determination

Clearly, the competent patient has a right to refuse treatment if that patient understands the consequences of such refusal, and no substantial state interests exist to override this right. The courts balance the competent patient's right to self-determination against state interests, which override the patient's right to refuse under certain circumstances. How this occurs will be discussed later in this text.

C. Policy Trend - Competent Patient

Abe Perlmutter was a 73-year-old man suffering from progressive, terminal amyotrophic lateral sclerosis. He was unable to move his extremities except for several fingers on one hand. At one time he had disconnected himself from his respiratory tubing; however, the alarms signaled the nurses to reconnect it. He asked that the machines be removed, and he be allowed to die. The physicians refused because they recognized that Florida law was not clear on the issue of disconnecting an artificial life-support system without being liable for homicide. The Florida Supreme Court reviewed the case in terms of compelling state interests. They found Mr. Perlmutter a competent individual. He had no minor dependents and his family members supported his desire to discontinue his life-prolonging treatment. The court finally held that Mr. Perlmutter's right to refuse treatment outweighed the state's interests, and ordered that his wishes be obeyed. The court cautioned, however, that its adoption of this principle was limited to the specific facts of this case. *Satz v. Perlmutter*, 379 So2d 359 (Fl 1980).

D. Compelling State Interests

1. Duty to preserve human life

The state has a paramount duty to preserve human life, particularly where that life has value to the person and society.

Appendix E:
ATLS
and the
Law

(Optional
Lecture)

2. Duty to protect innocent third party

The state has a duty to protect innocent third parties, such as children who are unable to make their own choices, and therefore may prevent a parent or guardian from exercising the right to refuse treatment on behalf of the minor.

3. Duty to prevent suicide

The state has a duty to prevent suicide. Preventing suicide must be distinguished from allowing patients to die from the natural course of a disease. Abe Perlmutter was not committing suicide when he requested that his advanced life-support systems be discontinued. He had no possible chance of recovery, and simply requested that nature take its course. Suicide is an act of specific intent in which the patient exercises his right to refuse treatment for a clearly reversible illness, solely to end his life.

4. Duty to help maintain the integrity of the medical profession

American courts are duly concerned that the right-to-refuse-treatment doctrine shall not be a "club" to coerce a physician either to abandon established medical therapy, or to become an "executioner." Where judges sense a compromise of medical integrity, they will either override the patient's right to refuse, or declare that the physician shall not be criminally liable.

E. State Interest Applied

1. Preschool vaccination

Preschool vaccination requirements have been validated by the Supreme Court, because no individual citizen has the right to jeopardize the health of the populace.

2. Court order to treat minors

The courts have ordered the treatment of minor children when parents have refused to permit them life-saving treatment.

3. Court order to an adult's guardian

The courts also have ordered blood transfusions for a retarded adult patient who was not terminally ill, and whose guardian had refused consent.

4. Court order to undergo treatment

Cases are on record in which the courts have ordered a competent adult to undergo treatment so that his or her minor children would not be denied the benefits of a supporting parent.

5. Court order to prevent deliberate suicide

A California court recently rejected the plea of a quadriplegic to be allowed to reject all nourishment and not be force-fed by hospital personnel. The court ruled that the state's interest in the preservation of life and

Appendix E:
ATLS
and the
Law

(Optional
Lecture)

the prevention of suicide outweighed the woman's desire to "die with dignity," because she would probably live another 15 to 20 years.

6. Court order to protect a fetus

An unusual case is on record in which a woman, pregnant with a viable fetus, was ordered to undergo a transfusion in order to protect the fetus.

VII. Artificial Life Support

A. Incompetent Patient/Substituted Judgment

The incompetent patient has the same substantive rights as the competent patient. The question is, how does the law protect the rights and fulfill the wishes of those who cannot act in their own behalf? The following cases demonstrate how the courts have either appointed a guardian to decide whether to terminate the artificial life-support system of an incompetent person, or have made that decision themselves. Many factors weigh in the court's decision in such cases. One factor is a clear and convincing statement by the patient, while competent, that he never wished to prolong his life by artificial means.

Another factor is the physical condition of the patient coupled with the physician's medical judgment regarding possibility of recovery. Finally, the wishes of the patient's family must be considered.

B. Legal Precedents

1. Quinlan case

The doctrine of substituted judgment is applied when a third party is allowed to step into the shoes of an incompetent patient. That third party may be the court, a natural guardian, or a court-appointed guardian. The famous Karen Quinlan case is an example of a situation in which the court appointed Karen's father as guardian, and allowed him to decide that her artificial life-support system should be discontinued. This case is also an example of the common-law doctrine that prevents one adult from exercising rights over another adult's body, whether competent or incompetent. Mr. Quinlan did not have the legal right to have the artificial life-support system discontinued until he was appointed the legal guardian of his adult, incompetent daughter. *In Re Quinlan*, 355 A2d 647 (1976).

2. Saikewicz case

The Saikewicz case is one example in which the court directly substituted its own judgment for that of the patient. A court will always presume that the patient wants his life extended, but the particular circumstances of Mr. Saikewicz's case overcame that presumption. In this case, the superintendent of Belchertown petitioned the court to appoint him the guardian of Mr. Saikewicz in order to prevent the patient from undergoing treatment for acute myelogenous leukemia. The court decided it was the best judge, and would have the greatest concern for Mr. Saikewicz, who was severely mentally retarded since birth.

**Appendix E:
ATLS
and the
Law**

**(Optional
Lecture)**

The court, as guardian, then decided that Mr. Saikewicz should not be forced to undergo treatment, because he was mentally incompetent and could not cooperate during the painful treatment process. Moreover, he would probably not live beyond six months, even with treatment.

This case caused a great deal of consternation in the medical profession, because the language of the decision implied that a physician would have to go to court in every case in which it was medically imprudent to treat a patient. *Supt. of Belchertown v. Saikewicz*, 370 NE2d 417 (1977). The Massachusetts court, however modified the Saikewicz decision in *Dinnerstein*.

3. Dinnerstein case

The Saikewicz case brought about the hospital's decision to petition the court concerning Shirley Dinnerstein, because the physician did not want to write a "do not resuscitate" (DNR) order for her. The court determined that Shirley Dinnerstein, a noncognitive, vegetative patient who was suffering from Alzheimer's disease, was in the terminal phase of a terminal illness. The court reasoned that a physician did not have to petition the court to write a DNR order if the patient suffered from an irreversible, noncognitive illness, and was in the terminal phase of that illness, provided the physician wrote the DNR order on the chart and wrote a progress note explaining his decision. The physician was also required to seek consultation from colleagues to substantiate his medical judgment. *Dinnerstein*, 380 NE2d 134 (1978).

C. Clear and Convincing Evidence

1. Legally brain-dead

A growing number of courts have adopted a clear-and-convincing-evidence doctrine to permit physicians to go beyond writing a DNR order, and to withdraw artificial life support altogether. When a patient is legally brain-dead, life has ended and there is no question that the law will permit physicians to withdraw artificial life support without fear of either criminal or civil prosecution. However, if the patient is brain-alive, a legal dilemma arises.

2. Eichner case

In the *Eichner* case, the treating physicians determined that clear and convincing evidence existed that while competent, the patient—now 83 years old and permanently vegetative—expressed a desire not to be coded or put on artificial life support. The New York court held that physicians can discontinue artificial life-support systems in such circumstances without fear of criminal or civil liability. The court went on to say that guardians of incompetent patients like Eichner were not required to petition the court to decide whether to discontinue life-support treatments. But should a disagreement arise among the treating physician, his colleagues, the family members of the patient, or other interested persons, the physician should always seek legal counsel in deciding whether to terminate life support. *In the Matter of Eichner* and *In the Matter of Storar*, 438 NYS2d 266 (1981).

**Appendix E:
ATLS
and the
Law**

**(Optional
Lecture)**

3. Right to die

Many states have responded to the dilemma of the brain-alive, incompetent patient by enacting statutes recognizing the right of individuals to privacy and dignity in establishing for themselves an appropriate level of medical care in specified medical situations. These "right-to-die" statutes provide a formal method by which a person can express his desire not to be put on artificial life support. However, euthanasia is never authorized by such laws.

D. Can Physicians Terminate Artificial Life Support?

In spite of cases like *Eichner* and "right-to-die" statutes, the law is still not completely clear with regard to the possible liability of a physician who discontinues the artificial life support for a patient in the terminal phase of a terminal illness, when the patient is brain-alive. In the *Eichner* case the patient was in a permanent vegetative state, and clear and convincing evidence was present that the patient would not have wanted artificial life support continued. If no such clear and convincing evidence exists, the physician has no clear mandate from the law to be allowed to terminate artificial life support in a situation in which medical judgment is clear, the family agrees, and a hospital ethics committee concurs. Some states have adopted this standard, but if a question exists concerning the solution to this dilemma, one should always seek legal guidance or even petition the court.

E. Policy Trend—Family Involvement

More and more courts, dealing with the problems of terminating artificial life support for an incompetent patient, recommend that the family be involved in such a decision. The courts are not clear as to whether they are changing the common-law doctrine regarding the ability of the next of kin to consent for the patient. Some speculate that the courts are suggesting family involvement in order to avoid civil and criminal lawsuits. In any event, the family of the patient, the hospital ethics committee, the treating physician, and his colleagues should all be in agreement that termination of artificial life support is the best solution for the patient before any action is even considered.

F. Can Physicians Stop a Code?

Physicians are involved daily in discontinuing CPR and advanced cardiac life support. Physicians should not rely solely on physical signs in deciding whether to discontinue CPR on a patient. The legal definition of death is now considered brain death, but brain death cannot be diagnosed during CPR because an EEG cannot be performed. The best measure of CPR failure in these situations is cardiac unresponsiveness. In the event that a physician is confronted in the emergency department with a sudden and unexpected death, a reasonable medical determination should be made that the patient is in the state of cardiac unresponsiveness. Only then should cardiac life support be discontinued. Judging from the standards noted in the cases presented here, the courts will accord great weight to the physician's medical judgment concerning when life has ceased.

G. Reasonable Medical Judgment

This discussion on "ATLS and the Law" is premised on the idea that in every circumstance, as much as possible, a physician will exercise reasonable medical judgment. Reasonable medical judgment means that the physician has considered the medical facts and has drawn a logical medical conclusion after exercising diligence and due care during the diagnostic and therapeutic processes. Where medical judgment is reasonable, it can and will be readily substantiated by a colleague. Reasonable medical judgment must precede all decisions not to treat or withdraw life support. The physician must not allow himself to become a philosopher, an ethicist, a moralist, or a sociologist prior to making a reasonable medical judgment that will withstand the scrutiny of his colleagues. The ethics committees and nonphysician decision-makers involved in such decisions must rely on the treating physician's reasonable medical judgment as the source for their decision to withdraw treatment or terminate life support.

VIII. Negligence

A. Elements

All negligence actions require that the plaintiff patient prove all four elements of negligence. The plaintiff must first establish the **standard of care** by expert medical testimony. Second, the plaintiff must establish a **breach** of that standard by the defendant physician. Third, the plaintiff must have a **demonstrable physical injury.** Fourth, the plaintiff must establish that the breach of duty was the logical and legal **cause** of the claimed injury.

B. Malpractice Claim

The plaintiff patient must show by a preponderance of the evidence (51% or a featherweight in the plaintiff's favor) that the defendant physician breached the standard of care applicable to the particular alleged malpractice claim, and that the breach of duty, legally and logically, caused the alleged injury.

C. Standard of Care

A physician has a legal duty to exercise that degree of knowledge, care, and skill that is expected of a reasonably competent practitioner in the same class in which he belongs, acting in the same or similar circumstances.

The key phrase in the standard of care, as defined by the courts, is **"in the same class in which he belongs."** This phrase would be a national standard enunciation if it referred to any specialist acting under the same or similar circumstances anywhere in the United States. For example, a member of a national society of dermatologists, whose members have met certain standards to belong to that society, will be held to the society's standards, regardless of where they practice. However, a small-town general practitioner in rural Idaho will typically not be held to the same standard as a general practitioner in New York City. The resources available to the two physicians are not comparable. However, available knowledge is comparable, especially the knowledge leading to the conclusion whether to transfer or refer the patient.

**Appendix E:
ATLS
and the
Law**

**(Optional
Lecture)**

The rule cited here is only a general rule, for some courts have held that certain aspects of medicine are so general in nature that English doctors may testify as expert witnesses as to those practices.

Other courts construe a standard of care whereby the physician will be compared to another physician who practices in the same geographic locality. In some states, a similarity rule even holds that the physician will be compared to another physician who practices in a similar locality under the same or similar circumstances. However, in those states, the presumption is that the similar locality may exist anywhere in the United States. The modern legal trend is moving toward a national standard of care, rather than one based strictly on regional or local practice.

Further, where a physician undertakes to treat a condition that would be referred to a specialist, the treating physician will be held to that standard of care required of the specialist. For example, a family practitioner was held to an orthopedic standard because he treated a comminuted fracture of the wrist that should have been referred to an orthopedist, or treated according to orthopedic standards. *Larsen v. Yelle,* 246 NW2d 841 (1976), Supreme Court of Minnesota.

D. ATLS Standard

A physician, rendering advanced trauma life support, has a legal duty to exercise that degree of knowledge, care, and skill expected of a reasonably competent physician trained in ATLS and acting in the same or similar circumstances.

The application of this standard is not based on right or wrong, but on what a reasonably competent ATLS physician would do under the circumstances of a particular case. For example, a patient appears in the emergency department after being flipped off a motorcycle, and has evidence of possible head and cervical spine injuries and shock. The ATLS physician has a duty to act reasonably, preventing further injury by properly immobilizing the patient's head and neck; obtaining crosstable, lateral cervical spine films; and initiating two large-caliber intravenous lines with Ringer's lactate. The physician is expected to make a reasonable assessment and act accordingly. He is not expected necessarily to make the absolute correct diagnosis at the time, but to support life until the correct diagnosis can be made and the patient transferred to a facility providing a higher level of care.

The standard of care does not require the physician to be correct in his initial diagnosis, but that he act reasonably under the circumstances of the case by providing the appropriate measures for advanced trauma life support.

IX. Summary

A. Physician/Patient Relationship

Physician/patient relationship has been discussed in terms of two legal theories, the mutual assent contract and undertaking to treat. The law will usually

**Appendix E:
ATLS
and the
Law**

**(Optional
Lecture)**

find a physician/patient relationship whenever a physician is involved in the treatment of a patient.

B. Consent

Consent arises from the law of battery. The importance of obtaining consent has been emphasized. However, the unlikelihood that informed consent will ever be an issue in advanced trauma life support also has been discussed.

C. Right to Refuse Treatment

The right to refuse treatment is a modern problem closely related to the principles of consent, and generally involves life-sustaining procedures. The competent patient has a right to refuse treatment. This right is based on the common-law doctrine of the right of privacy; the democratic principles of free choice; and the constitutional right against bodily invasion, as espoused by the Supreme Court. The state also has interests in this area that may outweigh the patient's right to refuse treatment.

D. Artificial Life Support

The issues surrounding the question of when to terminate the artificial life support of a terminally ill or vegetative, noncognitive patient have been reviewed.

E. Negligence

Legal negligence has been discussed. The four elements of negligence are: 1) duty—standard of care; 2) breach of duty—defendant physician acts negligently or negligently fails to act; 3) physical injury—the plaintiff must demonstrate a physical injury; and 4) causation—a plaintiff must demonstrate a logical and legal connection between the breach of duty and the alleged injury.

In summary, ATLS physicians must never operate under fear of the law. **Remember**, good medicine is good law. Whenever a physician acts reasonably under the circumstances of the case, exercising reasonable medical judgment, the likelihood is slim that a patient can bring a successful legal action against the physician.

Appendix F:
Organ and Tissue Donation

All patients should be considered initially as organ and/or tissue donors until they are ruled out for medical reasons. Cadaveric organ donors are previously healthy patients who have suffered irreversible, catastrophic brain injury of a known etiology, eg, brain trauma, subarachnoid hemorrhage, primary brain tumors, and cerebral anoxia. These patients can be any age. All solid organ donors should have intact cardiac function, and brain death should be confirmed by the number of physicians required by state law. Tissue donors do not require cardiac function.

Brain death is defined as irreversible cessation of brain function, including the cerebellum, brain stem, and first cervical vertebral segment. Brain death prevails in patients in whom other organ functions are maintained by artificial ventilation and pharmacological support. Brain death can be confirmed through apnea tests, electroencephalogram, and cerebral blood flow studies.

Contraindications for organ donation are insulin-dependent diabetes, systemic sepsis, autoimmune diseases, intravenous drug abuse, transmissible infections or disease, malignancy, sickle cell anemia, severe chronic hypertension, hepatitis, hemophilia, and homosexuality.

Organs and tissues that may be donated are:

1. Bone
2. Bone marrow
3. Corneas (eyes)
4. Skin
5. Soft tissues
6. Heart
7. Heart/lungs
8. Kidneys
9. Liver
10. Pancreas
11. Under special circumstances: intestines and endocrine tissue

Organ donation is covered in all 50 states of the United States by the Uniform Anatomical Gift Act (UAGA). The UAGA states that:

1. Persons over 18 years of age can donate.
2. Minors can donate with the consent of their parents.
3. The family of the deceased can donate organs.

Consent from the donor's relatives is obtained primarily through the use of a specifically drafted consent form. The UAGA also provides a method for securing relatives' consent through a recorded telephone conversation that must be witnessed by two or more people. However, discussion of the opportunity for organ donation is enhanced by direct contact with responsible relatives.

Donor referrals are usually accepted 24 hours a day, and potential donors can be discussed by contacting any active transplant service or organ procurement agency. Early referral is recommended in order to assess donor suitability, coordinate medicolegal requirements, initiate necessary lab tests, and to assure the complete collection of data.

Referrals can be expedited if the following patient data are available:

1. Patient history.

2. Diagnosis and date of admission.

3. ABO group.

4. Record of blood pressure and/or central venous pressure.

5. Fluid intake and output record.

6. Laboratory values, including BUN, creatinine, and urinalysis, etc.

7. Current medications.

8. Prehospital transport information.

Transplant physicians are usually available to assist with donor evaluation and donor maintenance, to discuss organ donation with next of kin, to perform donor surgery as necessary, to provide educational materials, and to coordinate the referral process.